Autism:
Behavior-Analytic Perspectives

Dedicated to

Larry, Carl, Sid,
Gary, Joe,
&
Jon

Autism:
Behavior-Analytic Perspectives

Edited by

Patrick M. Ghezzi

W. Larry Williams

James E. Carr

University of Nevada, Reno

CONTEXT PRESS
Reno, Nevada

iv

Autism: Behavior-Analytic Perspectives/ edited by Patrick M. Ghezzi, W. Larry
   Williams and James E. Carr.
   Includes bibliographical references

244 pp.   Hardback.   ISBN 1-878978-32-2

                 CIP #: RJ506.A9A898   1999
                         99-20586

Preface

The present volumn was developed from the proceedings of the Nevada Conference on Early Childhood Autism: Current Theory and Research. At the invitation of the editors, a small group of distinguished behavioral psychologists and educators gathered on the campus of the University of Nevada for several days in late January, 1998 to present and discuss among themselved their most recent conceptual and empirical work in early childhood autism. A small but spirited audience of students, teachers, and parents added to the mix to create the most stimulating working environment.

Each of the major presenters delivered a 45-minute paper, followed immediately by a 30-minute whole group discussion facilitated by a discussion leader. The chapters are lightly edited versions of those papers. The brief commentaries that follow each chapter were prepared by the designated discussion leader soon after the conference ended, and are intended to foster further analysis and elaboration.

We are confident that there is in this volumn, something for everyone with an avid interest in the theory, education, or treatment of children with autism. Readers will find that the science of behavior and behavior change dominates the collection of papers and commentaries, and for good reason: Behavior science has lead not only to a coherent understanding of autism, but also to a technology that is capable of forever altering those behaviors that are identified as autistic.

As this volumn attests, no one in the present group is resting on the laurels of their own work or of the science on which that work is based. Our understanding of autism is incomplete, and our technology is unfinished. As always, the outstanding challenges that lay ahead will be guided by the unfailing light of science. Leonardo da Vinci said it best when he wrote, "Those who fall in love with practice without science are like a sailor who enters a shipo without a helm or compass, and who never can be certain whither he is going."

We are grateful to Context Press and to the Unviersity of Nevada's Behavior analysis Program, the Department of Psychology, and the Graduate School for their support.

Patrick M. Ghezzi
W. Larry Williams
James E. Carr
February, 1999

Table of Contents

Chapter 1

Science and Ethics in
Early Intervention for Autism

Gina Green

New England Center for Children, E. K. Shriver Center for Mental Retardation, and Northeastern University

We propose that individuals who are recipients of treatment designed to change their behavior have the right to: (1) a therapeutic environment, (2) services whose overriding goal is personal welfare, (3) treatment by a competent behavior analyst, (4) programs that teach functional skills, (5) behavioral assessment and ongoing evaluation, and (6) the most effective treatment procedures available (Van Houten et al., 1988).

This summary of the position statement on "The Right to Effective Behavioral Treatment," adopted by the Executive Council of the Association for Behavior Analysis a decade ago, seems to me a fitting introduction to this paper and this conference. The position statement in its entirety is as good a summary of science-based, ethical practice standards for behavior analysts as any I have seen. It arose from controversies about therapeutic techniques derived from the science of behavior, in particular the use of aversive procedures. Its adoption did not make those controversies go away, of course, but the position statement did articulate standards for the effective and ethical delivery of behavioral interventions. For a time, it seemed that these standards influenced the behavior of many behavior analysts in ways that were adaptive for our discipline, and helped both behavior analysts and consumers of behavioral services resolve some of the controversies. Recently, many of those old controversies have resurfaced and some new ones have arisen in the arena of early intervention for autism. My observations from the "front lines" of these controversies suggest that it might be worthwhile to examine some of the burning scientific and ethical questions swirling around early behavioral intervention for autism within the framework of key points from the position statement.

I would like to start by discussing some of the challenges to science in general, and to behavior analysis in particular, presented by the current social and political milieu of autism treatment. In doing so I will attempt to illustrate some of the pseudoscientific and nonscientific practices that abound in mainstream autism treatment, examine some possible contributing factors, and discuss some implications. Then I will turn to some observations about practices within behavioral treatment for autism that bear a troubling resemblance to pseudoscience. Finally, I will offer some suggestions as to what behavior analysts can do to ensure that children with autism receive truly effective and ethical treatment.

Pseudoscience in Autism Treatment

I am going to assume that a detailed review of the essential elements of science is wholly unnecessary for this audience. Just to be sure that we start on the same page, however, and to help define what is **not** science, this is what I mean by "science," in a very oversimplified nutshell: The practice of science is the organized use of particular tools to put hunches or hypotheses to logical and empirical tests. The tools include (but are not limited to) operational definitions of the phenomena of interest; direct, accurate, reliable, and objective measurement; controlled experiments; reliance on data for drawing conclusions and making predictions; and replication of effects. These tools are wielded and their products are evaluated from a constantly skeptical perspective, one that does not take assertions or observations at face value, but seeks both proof of the occurrence of phenomena and the reasons for their occurrence. The goals of science are not to assume but to test, to seek not to confirm but to disconfirm hunches and beliefs. Good scientists take care to differentiate opinions, beliefs, and speculations from demonstrated facts; they don't make claims without supporting objective data.

In contrast, pseudoscience tries to lend credibility to beliefs, speculations, and untested assumptions by cloaking them in the accouterments of science—for example, by using scientific-sounding jargon, getting endorsements from individuals with apparent scientific credentials, perhaps even by using numbers or graphs. Pseudoscientific therapies for various conditions abound in today's culture. These therapies have several distinguishing features. They are often claimed to be extraordinarily effective, but that claim is not backed up with sound objective evidence. Testimonials, anecdotes, and personal accounts are offered instead. Risks such as negative side effects are rarely mentioned, or are downplayed. Information about the therapies is disseminated in materials published by promoters of the therapies, such as newsletters, videotapes, workshop handouts, books, advertisements, and more and more these days, Web pages. Purveyors of many of these therapies claim to have a secret formula or a mysterious, unique talent that renders them the only ones capable of delivering the therapy. At the same time, many of these therapies are claimed to be easy and quick, requiring little training or expertise. They are said to be effective for a wide range of problems or disorders (that is, they can cure whatever ails ya). There is an assumption that "new" or "innovative" equals "good"—that is, therapies that are new are automatically seen as better than "old" therapies. Promoters of pseudoscientific therapies are often working outside their areas of expertise. Some prescribe treatment over the phone, by mail, or via the Internet, without ever seeing the client in person. They don't conduct scientific studies, and they resist scrutiny and objective testing of their claims by others. Many offer their own training and "certification," a point to which I will return later (Green, 1996a; Randi, 1982; Sagan, 1995; Singer & Lalich, 1996).

Pseudoscience is everywhere these days. It has always been with us, but it is growing at an alarming rate, as evidenced by the increasing popularity of magical, mystical thinking, belief in the paranormal, and pursuit of nontraditional and unproved treatments for various disorders. It is also very big business. Millions of public and private dollars are spent on ineffective and bogus therapies each year. Then there are the thousands of dollars spent on attorney's fees and court costs when people who are harmed by pseudoscientific practices take legal action against the practitioners. For example, some very large monetary awards have been made to individuals who were harmed by practitioners of recovered memory therapy (Loftus & Ketcham, 1994; Singer & Lalich, 1996).

Autism treatment is a microcosm of the larger society in this respect. Since autism was first identified some 50 years ago, countless "breakthroughs" and "miracle cures" have been proclaimed. With each proclamation, hopes are raised dramatically. Precious resources are diverted from effective or potentially effective treatments to the latest "magic bullet." Whole new vocations and industries are spawned virtually overnight as self-declared experts take advantage of the desperation families feel to find a cure for autism. Some therapies enjoy great popularity for a while, only to be supplanted by the next fad that comes along. Some go dormant for a time, to be resurrected later. Many of these therapies for autism are said to be easy to use, readily available, rapidly and remarkably effective. Little or no training is required to implement them, or to evaluate whether they work. In fact, questions about whether, how, and why many of these therapies work are not even considered relevant, or at least are not to be addressed by accepted scientific methods. Faith and belief are all that's required. Rationales provided for some therapies for autism sound quite convincing, and many who promote them seem sincere and well-meaning. Often, however, those promoters are working outside their areas of expertise. Many therapies are based on flawed theories about the cause of autism, or on untested assumptions about the nature of the disorder. For the overwhelming majority of autism treatments, anecdotes and testimonials are the only supporting evidence. Almost none stand up to reasonably rigorous scientific evaluation. Indeed, many therapies for autism in widespread use today have been shown to be ineffective in scientific studies; some have even been shown to be harmful. Still others have not been subjected to any rigorous evaluations (Green, 1994, 1995, 1996a; Holmes, 1997; Klin & Cohen, 1997; Smith, 1993, 1996).

In short, many interventions for autism have all the earmarks of pseudoscience. The prototypic example, of course, is Facilitated Communication (FC), dubbed "the mother of all crazes in autism" by Wolfensberger (1994). This technique was claimed to enable thousands of individuals with autism and other disabilities to reveal previously hidden but precocious skills when "facilitators" held their hands or arms while together they pointed to letters to spell messages (e.g., Berger, 1992; Biklen, 1990, 1993; Crossley, 1992; Crossley & Remington-Gurney, 1992). When it was brought to North America from Australia in 1989, FC was hyped through self-published newsletters, books, videotapes, and media reports. It was claimed to be incredibly effective and easy to use (e.g., Berger, 1992; Biklen, 1990; Crossley, 1992). From the beginning, the promoters of FC resisted objective scrutiny and scientific testing (Biklen, 1990, 1993; DEAL, 1992). Their basic premise seemed to be that FC is such a fragile, ephemeral process that it evaporates upon testing. Essentially the same argument has been made, of course, by believers in ESP and other paranormal phenomena (Randi, 1982; Sagan, 1995). It was not surprising, then, that some FC proponents concluded that FC "proves" that many people with autism have ESP (Haskew & Donnellan, 1993).

Controlled studies of FC conducted in Australia in the late 1980s, and more than 30 published since, demonstrated that **facilitators** were the only ones who spelled reliably through FC, and that its use entailed such serious risks as the production of false accusations of sexual abuse, suppression of legitimate communications by people with disabilities, and inappropriate treatment decisions (Cummins & Prior, 1992; Green, 1994a, 1994b, 1995; Green & Shane, 1994; Hudson, 1995; Jacobson et al., 1994; Jacobson, Mulick, & Schwartz, 1995; Palfreman, 1994). There is not a scintilla of compelling objective evidence to support the claims about FC's effectiveness. Nevertheless, FC swept through substantial segments of the autism community like wildfire in the early '90s, and it continues to be used and promoted (e.g., Autism National Committee, 1995; Autism Society of America, 1995; Cardinal, Hanson, & Wakeham, 1996; Weiss, Wagner, & Bauman, 1996).

I review the FC phenomenon here to illustrate some important aspects of the mainstream autism culture. Many of the scientific and ethical questions we face about early behavioral intervention for autism must be considered in that context. To that end, it might be instructive to explore why pseudoscience flourishes in autism, while real science struggles to maintain a toehold. Why is it that FC and other pseudoscientific therapies garner widespread support, while applied behavior analysis is given short shrift? One thing my experiences with FC have taught me is never to underestimate the seductive power of "alternative" treatments and pseudoscience, for both consumers and promoters. Anything that promises to make a difficult situation easier and to make people feel better is tremendously appealing. It seems that when people feel bad, just doing **something** makes them feel better than doing nothing. When that something seems relatively easy, the person pushing it is warm and sincere and attentive, and it seems to produce an immediate effect, the operative contingencies are clear and the outcomes predictable. Skeptical observers of alternative healing practices have noted that many of these practitioners offer clients potent reinforcers, such as abundant attention, and get potent reinforcers in return, such as abundant fame and fortune (e.g., Randi, 1982; Singer & Lalich, 1996). In short, pseudoscientific pseudosolutions promise quick and easy relief from aversive conditions, and immediate positive reinforcement. Science, on the other hand, arrives at solutions to problems only slowly and methodically. It is no wonder that pseudoscience sells better than real science (Sagan, 1995; Tavris, 1997).

The autism culture has several features that make it especially fertile ground for pseudoscience. One contributing factor clearly is the severity and the mysterious nature of the disorder. Most parents receiving the diagnosis of autism for their child will be told it is a lifelong, severely disabling condition for which there is no cure and a generally poor prognosis (e.g., Cohen & Volkmar, 1997; Rapin, 1997). To say that this is a puzzling disorder that is extremely difficult to live with is a gross understatement. Those factors alone can lead families to reach out in desperation for anything and everything that might help. This desperation can create vulnerability to claims about quick fixes and miracle cures (Green, 1994, 1995, 1996a; Jacobson, Mulick, & Schwartz, 1995; Klin & Cohen, 1997; Maurice, 1993, 1996; Mulick, Jacobson, & Kobe, 1993). In my opinion, every professional who interacts with these families has a special responsibility to be sensitive to that vulnerability and to provide families with scientifically accurate information about autism and therapies for it. Unfortunately, however, even as therapies for autism proliferate at a dizzying rate, there seems to be a growing reluctance among professionals to provide families with sound, data-based guidance as to how to choose among them (cf. Green, 1996a; Maurice, 1993,1996).

To complicate matters further, most children with autism do not look disabled at all; in fact, many are strikingly attractive. Some seem to have astonishing special talents. These characteristics lend a mystique to autism, contributing to myths and magical thinking about the disorder. It's easy to believe that these are normal, even precocious, children who will reveal themselves only to the therapist or parent who has some sort of special intuition or technique. As Catherine Maurice (1993, 1996) has pointed out, this myth—the "hidden inner child"—has been part of the autism mystique since the disorder was first labeled. Not surprisingly, it originated in large part in the 1950s with that prototypic pseudoscientist, Bruno Bettelheim, who asserted that autism was a kind of severe emotional withdrawal caused by cold, rejecting parents. A recent biography revealed that Bettelheim not only fabricated his theory of autism out of whole cloth, he also claimed a remarkable "cure" rate for his own therapy for autism, but offered no credible evidence. Apparently Bettelheim fabricated his own credentials as well, claiming that he was trained in psychotherapy when in fact his only advanced degree was in art history (Pollak, 1997). But Bettelheim was a very skilled storyteller, and his views on autism were very convincing to many. They prevailed for at least three decades. This perhaps set the stage for the current state of affairs in autism: Theories and therapies gain favor on the strength of appealing stories and the personal repertoires of the storytellers, rather than hard data.

Pick up almost any popular newsletter or book on autism and you will probably notice a strong emphasis on personal accounts. Virtually anyone who is or was autistic, or who makes that claim, is granted expert status simply as a function of writing a book or making some speeches. If these individuals say that a treatment worked for them, many assume that the treatment ought to be used with others labeled autistic, regardless of any objective evidence about the treatment or the source. It is one thing for nonscientists to treat uncorroborated subjective reports as a basis for making treatment decisions, quite another when influential professionals do the same. Yet this is common in autism.

One other major contributor to the never-ending pursuit of unsubstantiated therapies in autism, in my opinion, is the "anything goes" stance of many professionals and organizations. The mainstream position is that there are many different treatment options. Consumers are encouraged to choose among them, without regard to objective evidence about their effectiveness or lack thereof (e.g., Autism Society of America Options Policy, 1997; but see Holmes, 1997). This amounts to an implicit endorsement of every fad treatment that comes down the pike. Such an approach is no more likely to produce lasting benefits for any individual with autism than it is to produce truly useful information about the disorder (Green, 1995, 1996a; Maurice, 1996).

All in all, it's not hard to see why pseudoscience and nonscience have always flourished in autism, while real science in general, and applied behavior analysis in particular, have not been well-received. These days, with more and more parents of children with autism seeking applied behavior analysis programming and refusing to settle for interventions that do not have comparable effectiveness, promoters of some other interventions seem to be stepping up their opposition to behavioral intervention. I have accompanied several parents to meetings with special education personnel in which the parents sought support for intensive behavioral programming. Often the parents have provided the educators with copies of all of the published outcome studies on early behavioral intervention for autism (see Green, 1996b for a review), as well as reviews of the hundreds of studies on behavioral intervention for autism that have accumulated since the 1960s (e.g., DeMyer, Hingtgen, & Jackson, 1981; Matson, Benavidez, Compton, Paclawskyj, & Baglio, 1996). In spite of that, I've heard behavioral intervention dismissed repeatedly by school personnel and their experts as "another fad treatment for autism," "experimental," and "just one of many options." The other "options" are typically touted as equally effective or superior to intensive behavioral intervention, but I have yet to see anyone produce sound supporting data. This brings up another factor that contributes to the ethical dilemmas some of us face: The federal special education law mandates that children with special needs receive an "appropriate" education, which has not always been construed to mean an effective education. Generally, public school personnel are free to choose the methods they use with children with autism; they are not required to use the most effective procedures available. Many families who seek intensive behavioral intervention for their young children with autism, however, have no choice but to turn to their local school district to provide that intervention or to pay for someone else to provide it. Unfortunately, this places many parents and their advocates in an adversarial position vis a vis the public education system (Williamson, 1996).

Recently I had the very unsettling experience of sitting front-and-center in a packed ballroom at the American Speech-Language-Hearing Association conference, listening to a presentation in which intensive behavioral intervention for autism and my own work were mischaracterized rather egregiously (Prizant & Wetherby, 1997). Next to me was a speech-language pathologist whose child with autism has benefited tremendously from intensive behavioral intervention. Both of us were dismayed when the presenters displayed a table from a recently published chapter listing several early intervention programs for children with autism, all reporting that about half of the children they serve end up in regular classrooms (Dawson & Osterling, 1997). The presenters did not point out that several of the programs listed in the table were based on applied behavior analysis to at least some extent, nor did they mention (until I asked) that few of those programs had published any comprehensive outcome data in the peer-reviewed scientific literature. The presenters' conclusion that all the various approaches represented in this table are as effective as intensive behavioral intervention was roundly applauded by the large audience. That experience told me a great deal about the strength of the "many options" credo and the uncritical acceptance of claims about interventions that characterize much of the autism culture today.

Pseudoscience in Behavior Analysis?

So far, I've spoken mostly about pseudoscientific practices outside of behavior analysis. Since behavior analysis is supposed to be a scientific discipline, I hope most behavior analysts would agree that pseudoscientific practices are unethical. Lately, however, I have observed some practices within the behavioral treatment of autism that look awfully like pseudoscience. To frame this discussion, I want to return to a portion of the "Right to Effective Behavioral Treatment" position statement. Item 6 states, "An individual has a right to the most effective treatment procedures available." It goes on to say,

An individual is entitled to effective and scientifically validated treatment. In turn, behavior analysts have an obligation to use only those techniques that have been demonstrated by researchers to be effective, to acquaint consumers and the public with the advantages and disadvantages of these techniques, and to search continuously for the most optimal means of changing behavior (Van Houten et al., 1988, p. 383).

Consider the phrases "most effective treatment procedures available" and "most optimal means of changing behavior" in light of the data we have in hand on intensive behavioral intervention for young children with autism. We have the 1987 study by Lovaas and the 1993 followup by McEachin, Smith and Lovaas reporting that a substantial proportion of children with autism who received intensive behavioral intervention (40 hours per week for at least 2 years) achieved normal functioning on several measures (e.g., IQ, language, challenging behavior, autistic characteristics, adaptive behavior, social behavior, school placement). Comparable control group children who received about 10 hours of behavioral intervention per week or standard nonbehavioral interventions made negligible, if any, gains over the same period of time. These studies are not perfect, as several reviewers have pointed out, but what study is? They raised many questions that need to be addressed in further research, and replications are sorely needed (e.g., Foxx, 1993; Green, 1996b; Gresham & MacMillan, 1997; Kazdin, 1993; Mesibov, 1993; Mundy, 1993; Schopler, Short, & Mesibov, 1989). Thankfully, at least one partial replication of the 1987 Lovaas study has been done by Birnbrauer and Leach (1993), with similar results. Additionally, there is corroborative evidence of the effectiveness of early intensive behavioral intervention in the form of the Princeton Child Development Institute's outcome study (Fenske et al., 1985), which predated the Lovaas study, and the case study on the Maurice children (Maurice, 1993; Perry, Cohen, & DeCarlo, 1995). The folks at PCDI have candidly acknowledged the limitations of their study, and I would be the last to say that we should base inferences about treatment effectiveness on uncontrolled studies alone. I want to say for the record, however, that I have now known the two Maurice children for nearly four years. In addition to interacting with them a good deal, I've seen the data on their original diagnoses, numerous school reports from teachers who know nothing of their histories, and some of their standardized academic achievement test scores. I have no doubts about either the validity of their autism diagnosis or their complete recovery from autism. They are normal, bright, very verbal, creative, sensitive, and loving children.

Now to return to the published evidence on early intensive behavioral intervention for autism. It has been the subject of heated criticism, some justified, some not, in my opinion. Despite the limitations of the current research, however, it seems to me that early intensive behavioral intervention for autism meets the standard of "most effective treatment procedures available" specified in the ABA position statement (VanHouten et al., 1988). I base this conclusion on the following:

(1) Several longitudinal studies of cohorts of individuals with autism found that very few improved substantially as a result of participating in generic special education and other therapies (e.g., Eaves & Ho, 1996; Freeman, Ritvo, Needleman, & Yokota, 1985; Freeman et al., 1991).

(2) No interventions for autism except applied behavior analysis are currently supported by sound scientific evidence that they reliably produce large, comprehensive, and lasting improvements (Green, 1996a; Schreibman, 1993; Smith, 1993, 1996).

(3) There is suggestive evidence that less intensive early behavioral intervention does not produce improvements as large as those documented to result from intensive intervention (Anderson, Avery, DiPietro, Edwards, & Christian, 1987; Lovaas, 1987).

(4) Unless I have missed it despite diligent searching, there is no evidence in the peer-reviewed scientific literature that other, less intensive behavior analysis approaches produce long-term outcomes comparable to the intensive approach (but perhaps some of the other presenters at this conference will enlighten us to the contrary).

Despite this evidence, I am aware that a number of behavior analysts expressly and actively oppose early intensive behavioral intervention for autism. They testify in special education due process hearings and court cases against families seeking intensive behavioral intervention, recommend other approaches in written evaluations, and advise parents, schools, other professionals, and policymakers not to support early intensive behavioral intervention. I am well aware that some of these behavior analysts must operate under constraining political and financial contingencies, and I can understand why some would opt to behave cautiously until more data are in. I find it troubling, however, that some behavior analysts refuse to credit the notion that early intensive behavioral intervention can produce normal functioning in some children. It is certainly difficult to explain that to the many parents of young children with autism who expect behavior analysts, of all people, to stand on the best available scientific evidence.

Another item in the "Right to Effective Treatment" statement says, "An individual has a right to treatment by a competent behavior analyst." One of the questions I hear most often from parents, schools, insurance companies, and policymakers is, "How do we know if someone is competent to provide applied behavior analysis services to children with autism?" With the market for these services growing, a lot of opportunists are claiming falsely to be competent behavior analysts. To complicate matters further, apparently some individuals and groups have stated that they are "certifying" professionals in the behavioral treatment of autism, or in the use of some behavioral techniques or methods, outside of any legally established credentialling process (e.g., Buch, 1996). In their recent book "Crazy Therapies," Margaret Thaler Singer and Janja Lalich (1996) make the following point about pseudoscientific therapies, which I think those who would undertake to do their own "certification" might do well to ponder:

> . . . One marketing technique that has done well in the professional world is to start a certification program . . . Being able to display an award with a gold embossed seal stating that the holder is "certified" has apparently clinched the deal on many workshops and programs. The public is led to think that some higher, socially approved agency has awarded the certificate. The certifiers ride on the tails of state licensure, as well as on the aura of sanctity and credibility of state medical boards, . . . boards of examiners, famous universities, or other legally sanctioned agencies whose stamp of approval typically means that some minimum standards have been met. . . . Sometimes only one man or woman is the total organization issuing the certificates. We're not saying that the multitude of organizations offering certification are all phony or illegal, but we want to call attention to the remarkable propaganda value such a piece of paper appears to carry in the public eye. (pp.167-168)

On a related note, I've heard and seen several statements implying strongly that there is only one program that can provide, and train people to provide, effective behavioral intervention for children with autism (e.g., Buch, 1996; Families for Intensive Autism Treatment, 1996; State of Wisconsin, 1997). To me, that suggests that there is some mysterious, idiosyncratic formula for behavioral intervention, and that only one program has the recipe. Clearly, some very special skills are required to provide behavioral intervention to children with autism, in particular to direct and supervise programming for a number of children competently and ethically. But there's nothing magical or mysterious about those skills. A number of people have them and a number of universities and programs teach them (although not nearly enough). No one holds a patent or copyright on those skills or the large body of knowledge on which they are based. Those who reinforce the notion that a single person or program has a "secret recipe" for the behavioral treatment of autism should not be surprised when others accuse them of engaging in guru worship and other pseudoscientific practices. That is precisely what is happening today, and if it continues, it will hurt behavior analysis as well as children with autism and their families sooner or later.

Over the past four years or so, I have had many opportunities to observe firsthand various programs for children with autism that were described as "behavioral" or "behavior analytic." Some were home-based, some were in private schools or centers, and still others were in public schools. Many were very good: The individuals working directly with the children had excellent behavioral teaching skills, were enthusiastic and positive in their interactions with children, and used objective data to evaluate children's progress continuously and adjust programming accordingly. Many of these individuals were parents who had become outstanding behavior change agents. Children received high rates of rapidly paced learning opportunities, arranged in both discrete-trial and incidental teaching formats. There was very little "down" time. The main approach to reducing problem behavior was skill-building with positive reinforcement. Each child had an individualized curriculum guided by an overall scope-and-sequence of skills based on typical development, and broken down into components. Intensive training in "learning to learn," communication, academic, play, and social skills had high priority. Most of the good programs I have seen were directed by people with advanced formal training in behavior analysis and considerable experience in working intensively with youngsters with autism. Some programs incorporated many of the best available techniques from the current behavior analysis literature—although I have to say that even the best could do better in such areas as teaching various kinds of discrimination skills. There is a rich technology for teaching simple and conditional discriminations and stimulus equivalence to learners with disabilities that simply has not made its way from research into practice (e.g., Cowley, Green, & Braunling-McMorrow, 1992; Dixon, 1981; Dixon, Dixon, & Spradlin, 1983; Dube, Iennaco, & McIlvane, 1993; Dube, Iennaco, Rocco, Kledaras, & McIlvane, 1992; Dube, McDonald, McIlvane, & Mackay, 1991; Green, 1990, 1993; Kelly, Green, & Sidman, 1998; Mackay, 1985, 1991; Mackay & Sidman, 1984; McDonagh, McIlvane, & Stoddard, 1984; McIlvane, Dube, Green, & Serna, 1992; Saunders & Spradlin, 1989, 1993; Sidman, 1971, 1977; Sidman & Stoddard, 1967; Spradlin, Cotter, & Baxley, 1973; Stoddard, Bradley & McIlvane, 1987; Stoddard, Brown, Hurlbert, Manoli, & McIlvane, 1989; Stromer, 1991; Stromer & Mackay, 1992, 1993; Zygmont, Lazar, Dube, & McIlvane, 1992). My guess is that the good programs would be even better if they used some of that technology.

Unfortunately, many other programs I've observed had few of the features I just described. They incorporated none of the many techniques that recent research has shown to be effective for teaching children with autism—techniques that minimize errors and reduce prompt dependency, enhance generalization, and promote communication, for example. Other techniques that have not been validated scientifically, however, were being used in some of these programs, such as sensory integration therapy, auditory integration training, special diets, and the like (see Green, 1996a; Smith, 1993, 1996) No real data were being collected; instead, subjective impressions recorded in anecdotal notes were used to evaluate children's progress. There was no analysis of either learning difficulties or problem behavior; procedures were simply applied in cookbook fashion. If they didn't work they were just abandoned and replaced with other procedures, or the child or parents were blamed. In many cases those delivering the intervention were not well-trained or supervised; no one with advanced training and experience directly observed the children or the therapists more often than once every 3-6 months. In fact, no one with advanced training and experience was involved at all in many instances; the programs were directed entirely by individuals with bachelor's degrees or less, some of whom charged exorbitant fees. The serious implications of these practices for children with autism and for our field should be obvious.

Some Recommendations

What can behavior analysts do to resolve some of the scientific and ethical controversies about early intervention for autism? How can we avoid the pitfalls of pseudoscience? I have a few specific suggestions.

First and foremost, it should go without saying that we need to **get more data**. One of the highest priorities for behavior analysts involved in early intervention for autism should be sound research to address the many scientific and practical questions raised by the studies of early intensive behavioral intervention (Anderson et al., 1987; Birnbrauer & Leach, 1993; Fenske et al.,1985; Graff, Green, & Libby, 1998; Lovaas, 1987; McEachin, Smith, & Lovaas, 1993; Smith, Eikeseth, Klevstrand, & Lovaas, 1997). We need operational definitions of intensive treatment, measures of treatment integrity, data on child characteristics that relate to treatment responsiveness, measures of social validity, comparisons of different levels of intensive treatment, and comparisons of intensive behavioral intervention with other "brands" of applied behavior analysis and with nonbehavioral interventions, to give just a few examples. All of us who are involved in early intervention for autism need to document short- and long-term outcomes in ways that will be convincing not only to our colleagues, but to other scientists and the public. Cost-benefit analyses are also needed. John Jacobson, Jim Mulick, and I have undertaken one analysis of the potential costs and savings of early intensive behavioral intervention, but again, comparisons with other behavioral and nonbehavioral approaches would be informative (Jacobson, Mulick, & Green, in press).

Second, we need to try to reduce the polarization that is developing among some behavior analysts around early intensive behavioral intervention for autism. It would be best to resolve those differences on the basis of data, rather than politics and personal repertoires. We have been presented with some golden opportunities to advance both behavior analysis and autism research significantly. Let's focus on our common goals, and on the best interests of the children and their families.

Third, I personally would like to see all applied behavior analysts renew their vows, so to speak, with science. I fear that if the practice of behavior analysis drifts away from science, we will find ourselves in the same situation as psychology did not too long ago. Behavior analysis simply cannot afford a major rift between scientists and practitioners, in autism treatment or any other area. Perhaps it is time for the field to revive, or at least revisit, the "Right to Effective Behavioral Treatment" position statement (VanHouten et al., 1988).

Fourth, I believe it is past time for behavior analysis to adopt some kind of wide-scale, formal procedures for certifying practitioners (like the procedures in place in Florida, for instance; Shook & Favell, 1996; Shook, 1993; Shook, Hartsfield, & Hemingway, 1995). Efforts are underway in some states as we speak, spurred in part by some of the things that are happening in early autism intervention. Certification needs to be done carefully, however, to provide both consumers of behavioral services and our discipline with appropriate safeguards. Otherwise we run the risk of falling into some of the pseudoscientific traps I mentioned earlier.

Finally, I challenge behavior analysts to speak up about pseudoscience and nonscience in autism and elsewhere. Failing to point out to parents and others that a therapy for autism has no scientific or logical support is tantamount to reinforcing pseudoscience and perpetuating the endless cycle of false hopes and bogus therapies. Many colleagues have told me that they don't speak up about unproved and ineffective therapies because they don't want to burst bubbles, or they don't want to seem impolite. To that I say, the truth isn't always pretty or pleasant, but it's always the truth. Better to reveal it sooner than later. Many consumers are looking for someone—anyone—to tell them the truth about the scientific evidence for and against various treatments for autism. Behavior analysts are supposed to be scientists. If not us, who?

References

Anderson, S.R., Avery, D.L., DiPietro, E.K., Edwards, G.L., & Christian, W.P. (1987). Intensive home-based early intervention with autistic children. *Education and Treatment of Children, 10*, 352-366.

Autism National Committee (1995). *The Communicator*, Vol. 6, No. 2.

Autism Society of America (1995). *Advocate*, Jan. - Feb.

Autism Society of America (1997). ASA Options Policy. *Advocate, 29*, 4.

Berger, C. (1992). Experiences with Facilitated Communication: The breakthrough. *The Advocate, Fall*, 17-18.

Biklen, D. (1990). Communication unbound: Autism and praxis. *Harvard Educational Review, 60*, 291-315.

Biklen, D. (1993). *Communication unbound: How facilitated communication is challenging traditional views of autism and ability-disability.* New York: Teachers College Press.

Birnbrauer, J.S., & Leach, D.J. (1993). The Murdoch early intervention program after 2 years. *Behaviour Change, 10*, 63-74.

Buch, G. (1996, November). *Professional and research issues in early behavioral intervention.* Paper presented at the meeting of the Kansas Autism Society, Kansas City.

Cardinal, D.N., Hanson, D., & Wakeham. (1996). Investigation of authorship in Facilitated Communication. *Mental Retardation, 34,* 231-242.

Cohen, D.J., & Volkmar, F.R. (1997*). Handbook of autism and pervasive developmental disorders.* New York: John Wiley & Sons.

Cowley, B.J., Green, G., & Braunling-McMorrow, D. (1992). Using stimulus equivalence procedures to teach name-face matching to adults with brain injuries. *Journal of Applied Behavior Analysis, 25,* 461-475.

Crossley, R. (1992). Getting the words out: Case studies in facilitated communication training. *Topics in Language Disorders, 12,* 46-59.

Crossley, R., & Remington-Gurney, J. (1992). Getting the words out: Facilitated communication training. *Topics in Language Disorders, 12,* 29-45.

Cummins, R.A., & Prior, M.P. (1992). Autism and assisted communication: A response to Biklen. *Harvard Educational Review, 62,* 228-241.

Dawson, G., & Osterling, J. (1997). Early intervention in autism. In M.J. Guralnick (Ed.), *The effectiveness of early intervention: Second generation research.* Baltimore: Paul H. Brookes.

DEAL Communication Centre (1992). *Facilitated communication training.* Melbourne, Australia: Author.

DeMyer, M.K., Hingtgen, J.N., & Jackson, R.K. (1981). Infantile autism reviewed: A decade of research. *Schizophrenia Bulletin, 7,* 388-451.

Dixon, L.S. (1981). A functional analysis of photo-object matching skills of severely retarded adolescents. *Journal of Applied Behavior Analysis, 14,* 465-478.

Dixon, M.H., Dixon, L.S., & Spradlin, J.E. (1983). Analyses of individual differences of stimulus control among developmentally disabled children. *Advances in Learning and Behavioral Disabilities, 2,* 85-110.

Dube, W.V., Iennaco, F.M., & McIlvane, W.J. (1993). Generalized identity matching to sample of two-dimension forms in individuals with intellectual disabilities. *Research in Developmental Disabilities, 14,* 457-477.

Dube, W.V., Iennaco, F.M., Rocco, F.J., Kledaras, J.B., & McIlvane, W.J. (1992). Microcomputer-based programmed instruction in generalized identity matching for persons with severe disabilities. *Journal of Behavioral Education, 2,* 29-51.

Dube, W.V., McDonald, S.J., McIlvane, W.J., & Mackay, H.A. (1991). Constructed-response matching to sample and spelling instruction. *Journal of Applied Behavior Analysis, 24,* 305-317.

Eaves, L.C., & Ho, H.H. (1996). Brief report: Stability and change in cognitive and behavioral characteristics of autism through childhood. *Journal of Autism and Developmental Disorders, 26,* 557-569.

Families for Intensive Autism Treatment (1996). Service providers. *FIAT Newsletter, 2,* 2.

Fenske, E.C., Zalenski, S., Krantz, P.J., & McClannahan, L.E. (1985). Age at intervention and treatment outcome for autistic children in a comprehensive intervention program. *Analysis and Intervention in Developmental Disabilities, 5,* 49-58.

Foxx, R.M. (1993). Sapid effects awaiting independent replication. *American Journal on Mental Retardation, 97,* 375-376.

Freeman, B.J., Rahbar, B., Ritvo, E.R., Bice, T.L., Yokota, A., & Ritvo, R. (1991). The stability of cognitive and behavioral paramters in autism: A twelve-year prospective study. *Journal of the American Academy of Child and Adoelscent Psychiatry, 30*, 479-482.

Freeman, B.J., Ritvo, E.R., Needleman, R., & Yokota, A. (1985). The stability of cognitive and linguistic parameters in autism: A five-year prospective study. *Journal of the American Academy of Child Psychiatry, 24*, 459-464.

Graff, R.B., Green, G., & Libby, M.E. (1998). Effects of two levels of treatment intensity on a young child with severe disabilities. *Behavioral Interventions, 13*, 21-41.

Green, G. (1990). Differences in development of visual and auditory-visual equivalence relations. *American Journal on Mental Retardation, 95*, 260-270.

Green, G. (1993). Stimulus control technology for teaching number/quantity equivalences. *Proceedings of the 1992 National Autism Conference (Australia)*. Melbourne, Victoria, Australia: Victorian Autistic Children's and Adults' Association.

Green, G. (1994). The quality of the evidence. In H.C. Shane (Ed.), *Facilitated Communication: The clinical and social phenomenon* (pp. 157-225). San Diego: Singular Publishing.

Green, G. (1994). Facilitated Communication: Mental miracle or sleight of hand? *Skeptic, 2*, 68-76; reprinted (1994) *Behavior and Social Issues, 4*, 69-85.

Green, G. (1995). An ecobehavioral interpretation of the Facilitated Communication phenomenon. *Psychology in Mental Retardation and Developmental Disabilities, 21*, 1-8.

Green, G. (1996a). Evaluating claims about treatments for autism. In C. Maurice, G. Green, & S. Luce (Eds.), *Behavioral intervention for young children with autism: A manual for parents and professionals* (pp. 15-28). Austin, TX: PRO-ED.

Green, G. (1996b). Early behavioral intervention for autism: What does research tell us? In C. Maurice, G. Green, & S. Luce (Eds.), *Behavioral intervention for young children with autism: A manual for parents and professionals (pp. 29-44)*. Austin, TX: PRO-ED.

Green, G., & Shane, H.C. (1994). Science, reason, and Facilitated Communication. *Journal of the Association for Persons with Severe Handicaps, 19*, 151-172.

Gresham, F.M., & MacMillan, D.L. (1997). Autistic recovery? An analysis and critique of the empirical evidence on the early intervention project. *Behavioral Disorders, 22*, 185-201.

Haskew, P., & Donnellan, A.M. (1992). *Emotional maturity and well-being: Psychological lessons of facilitated communication.* Danbury, CT: DRI Press.

Holmes, D.L. (1997). Prologue to guidelines for theories and practices. *Advocate, 29*, 9-10.

Hudson, A. (1995). Disability and facilitated communication: A critique. In T.H. Ollendick & R.J. Prinz (Eds.), *Advances in Clinical Child Psychology* (Vol. 1, pp. 95-107), New York: Plenum Press.

Jacobson, J.W., Eberlin, M., Mulick, J.A., Schwartz, A.A., Szempruch, J., & Wheeler, D.L. (1994). Autism and Facilitated Communication: Future directions. In J.L.

Matson (Ed.), *Autism in children and adults: Etiology, diagnosis, and treatment.* (pp. 59-83). Pacific Grove, CA: Brooks/Cole.

Jacobson, J.W., Mulick, J.A., & Green, G. (in press). Cost-benefit estimates for early intensive behavioral intervention for young children with autism: General model and single state case. *Behavioral Interventions.*

Jacobson, J.W., Mulick, J.A., & Schwartz, A.A. (1995). A history of Facilitated Communication: Science, pseudoscience, and antiscience. *American Psychologist, 50,* 750-765.

Kazdin, A.E. (1993). Replication and extension of behavioral treatment of autistic disorder. *American Journal on Mental Retardation, 97,* 377-379.

Kelly, S., Green, G., & Sidman, M. (1998). Visual identity matching and auditory-visual matching: A procedural note. *Journal of Applied Behavior Analysis, 31,* 237-243.

Klin, A., & Cohen, D.J. (1997). Ethical issues in research and treatment. In D.J. Cohen & F. R. Volkmar (Eds.), *Handbook of autism and pervasive developmental disorders* (pp. 828-841). New York: John Wiley & Sons.

Loftus, E., & Ketcham, K. (1994). *The myth of repressed memory.* New York: St. Martin's Griffin.

Lovaas, O.I. (1987) Behavioral treatment and normal educational and intellectual functioning in young autistic children. *Journal of Consulting and Clinical Psychology, 55,* 3-9.

Mackay, H. A. (1985). Stimulus equivalence in rudimentary reading and spelling. *Analysis and Intervention in Developmental Disabilities, 5,* 373-387.

Mackay, H. A. (1991). Stimulus equivalence: Implications for the development of adaptive behavior. In B. Remington (Ed.), *The challenge of severe mental handicap* (pp. 235-259). New York: Wiley.

Mackay, H. A., & Sidman, M. (1984). Teaching new behavior via equivalence relations. In P. H. Brooks, R. Sperber, & C. McCauley (Eds.), *Learning and cognition in the mentally retarded* (pp. 493-513). Hillsdale, NJ: Erlbaum.

Matson, J.L., Benavidez, D.A., Compton, L.S., Paclawskyj, T., & Baglio, C. (1996). Behavioral treatment of autistic persons: A review of research from 1980 to the present. *Research in Developmental Disabilities, 17,* 433-465.

Maurice, C. (1993). *Let me hear your voice.* New York: Knopf.

Maurice, C. (1996). Why this manual?. In C. Maurice (Ed.), G. Green, & S.C. Luce (Co-Eds.), *Behavioral intervention for young children with autism: A manual for parents and professionals* (pp. 3-12). Austin, TX: PRO-ED.

McDonagh, E. C., McIlvane, W. J., & Stoddard, L. T. (1984). Teaching coin equivalences via matching to sample. *Applied Research in Mental Retardation, 5,* 177-197.

McEachin, J.J., Smith, T., & Lovaas, O.I. (1993). Long-term outcome for children with autism who received early intensive behavioral treatment. *American Journal on Mental Retardation, 4,* 359-372.

McIlvane, W. J., Dube, W. V., Green, G., & Serna, R. W. (1993). Programming conceptual and communication skill development: A methodological stimulus-class analysis. In A. P. Kaiser &D. B. Gray (Eds.), *Enhancing children's communication: Research foundations for intervention* (pp. 243-285). Baltimore: Brooks.

Mesibov, G.B. (1993). Treatment outcome is encouraging. *American Journal on Mental Retardation, 97*, 379-380.

Mulick, J.A., Jacobson, J.W., & Kobe, R.H. (1993). Anguished silence and helping hands: Miracles in autism with Facilitated Communication. *Skeptical Inquirer, 17*, 270-280.

Mundy, P. (1993). Normal versus high-functioning status in children with autism. *American Journal on Mental Retardation, 97*, 381-384.

Palfreman, J. (1994). The Australian origins of Facilitated Communication. In H.C. Shane (Ed.), *Facilitated Communication: The clinical and social phenomenon.* (pp. 33-56). San Diego: Singular Publishing.

Perry, R., Cohen, I., & DeCarlo, R. (1995). Case study: Deterioration, autism, and recovery in two siblings. *Journal of the American Academy of Child and Adolescent Psychiatry, 34*, 232-237.

Pollak, R. (1997). *The creation of Dr. B.* New York: Simon & Schuster.

Prizant, B. M., & Wetherby, A.M. (1997, November). *Treatment approaches for young children with pervasive developmental disorders: A critical review.* Paper presented at the annual conference of the American Speech-Language-Hearing Association, Boston.

Randi, J. (1982). *Flim-flam!* Buffalo, NY: Prometheus Books.

Rapin, I. (1997). Autism. *The New England Journal of Medicine, 337*, 97-104.

Sagan, C. (1995). *The demon-haunted world: Science as a candle in the dark.* New York: Random House.

Saunders, K. J., & Spradlin, J. E. (1989). Conditional discrimination in mentally retarded adults: The effect of training the component simple discriminations. *Journal of the Experimental Analysis of Behavior, 52*, 1-12.

Saunders, K. J., & Spradlin, J. E. (1993). Conditional discrimination in mentally retarded subjects: Programming acquisition and learning set. *Journal of the Experimental Analysis of Behavior, 60*, 571-585.

Schopler, E., Short, A., & Mesibov, G. (1989). Relation of behavioral treatment to "normal functioning": Comment on Lovaas. *Journal of Consulting and Clinical Psychology, 57*, 162-164.

Schreibman, L. (1988). *Autism.* Newbury Park, CA: Sage.

Shook, G.L. (1993). The professional credential in behavior anlaysis. *The Behavior Analyst, 16*, 87-101.

Shook G.L., & Favell, J.E. (1996). Identifying qualified professionals in behavior analysis. In C. Maurice, G. Green, & S.C. Luce (Eds.), *Behavioral intervention for young children with autism: A manual for parents and professionals* (pp. 221-229). Austin, TX: PRO-ED.

Shook, G.L., Hartsfield, F., & Hemingway, M. (1995). Essential content for training behavior analysis practitioners. *The Behavior Analyst, 18,* 83-92.

Sidman, M. (1971). Reading and auditory-visual equivalences. *Journal of Speech and Hearing Research, 14,* 5-13.

Sidman, M. (1977). Teaching some basic prerequisites for reading. In P. Mittler (Ed.), *Research to practice in mental retardation Vol. 2: Education and training* (pp. 353-360). Baltimore, MD: University Park Press.

Sidman, M., & Cresson, O., Jr. (1973). Reading and crossmodal transfer of stimulus equivalences in severe retardation. *American Journal of Mental Deficiency, 77,* 515-523.

Sidman, M., & Stoddard, L.T. (1967). The effectiveness of fading in programming a simultaneous form discrimination for retarded children. *Journal of the Experimental Analysis of Behavior, 10,* 3-15.

Singer, M.T., & Lalich, J. (1996). *"Crazy" therapies.* San Francisco: Jossey-Bass.

Smith, T. (1993). Autism. In T.R. Giles (Ed.), *Handbook of effective psychotherapy* (pp. 107-133). New York: Plenum.

Smith, R. (1996). Are other treatments effective? In C. Maurice, G. Green, & S.C. Luce (Eds.), *Behavioral intervention for young children with autism: A manual for parents and professionals* (pp. 45-59). Austin, TX: PRO-ED.

Smith, R., Eikeseth, S., Klevstrand, M., & Lovaas, O.I. (1997). Intensive behavioral treatment for preschoolers with severe mental retardation and pervasive developmental disorders. *American Journal on Mental Retardation, 102,* 238-249.

Spradlin, J. E., Cotter, V. W., & Baxley, N. (1973). Establishing a conditional discrimination without direct training: A study of transfer with retarded adolescents. *American Journal of Mental Deficiency, 77,* 556-566.

State of Wisconsin (1997). *Bureau of Health Care Financing Medicaid Prior Authorization Guidelines, Intensive In-home Autism Services.*

Stoddard, L. T., Bradley, D. P., & McIlvane, W. J. (1987). Stimulus control of emergent performances: Teaching money skills. In J. A. Mulick & R. F. Antonak (Eds.), *Transitions in mental retardation: Vol. 2. Issues in therapeutic intervention* (pp. 113-149). Norwood, NJ: Ablex.

Stoddard, L. T., Brown, J., Hurlbert, B., Manoli, C., & McIlvane, W. J. (1989). Teaching money skills through stimulus class formation, exclusion, and component matching methods: Three case studies. *Research in Developmental Disabilities, 10,* 413-439.

Stromer, R. (1991). Stimulus equivalence: Implications for teaching. In W. Ishaq (Ed.), *Human behavior in today's world* (pp. 109-122). NY: Praeger Publishers.

Stromer, R., & Mackay, H.A. (1992). Delayed constructed-response identity matching improves the spelling performance of students with mental retardation. *Journal of Behavioral Education, 2,* 139-156.

Stromer, R., & Mackay, H.A. (1993). Delayed identity matching to complex samples: Teaching students with mental retardation spelling and the prerequisites for equivalence classes. *Research in Developmental Disabilities, 14,* 19-38.

Tavris, C. (June, 1997). *Back to rationality: The science and politics of gender research.* Paper presented at the meeting of the Rational Feminist Alliance of the Committee for the Scientific Investigation of Claims of the Paranormal (CSICOP), Boulder, CO.

VanHouten, R., Axelrod, S., Bailey, J.S., Favell, J.E., Foxx, R.M., Iwata, B.A., & Lovaas, O.I. (1988). The right to effective behavioral treatment. *Journal of Applied Behavior Analysis, 21*, 381-384.

Weiss, M.J.S., Wagner, S.H., & Bauman, M.L. (1996). A validated case study of Facilitated Communication. *Mental Retardation, 34*, 220-230.

Williamson, M. (1996). Funding the behavioral program: Legal strategies for parents. In C. Maurice, G. Green, & S.C. Luce (Eds.), *Behavioral intervention for young children with autism: A manual for parents and professionals* (pp. 267-293). Austin, TX: PRO-ED.

Wolfensberger, W. (1994). The Facilitated Communication "craze" as an instance of pathological science: The cold fusion of human services. In H.C. Shane (Ed.), *Facilitated Communication: The clinical and social phenomenon* (pp. 57-122) San Diego: Singular Press.

Zygmont, D. M., Lazar, R. M., Dube, W. V., & McIlvane, W. J. (1992). Teaching arbitrary matching via sample stimulus-control shaping to young children and mentally retarded individuals: A methodological note. *Journal of the Experimental Analysis of Behavior, 57,* 109-117.

Discussion of Green

Data Are Not Enough

Jane S. Howard
California State University, Stanislaus

The Problem

As Green (this volume) notes, when adoption is the dependent measure, pseudoscience often trumps science. The problem is not unique to autism, behavior analysis, or even this time and place. Consider Project Follow Through.

Project Follow Through, the most extensive (and expensive) study of effective educational practices ever undertaken in the world, identified Direct Instruction as the most efficacious solution for teaching "at risk" kindergarten and elementary school children. Begun in 1968, Project Follow Through was funded by the federal government and involved more than 200,000 children and almost $1,000,000,000. The resulting data generated controversy as almost all of the educational models, with the exception of Direct Instruction, were remarkably ineffective (The Behavior Analytic Model generally ranked second in effectiveness.) Moreover, the data also showed that children participating in many of the models (especially the ones which emphasized affective domains) fared less well academically than they would have if they had not received the "benefit" of these Follow Through dollars.

The purported objective of Project Follow Through was to disseminate effective models to the public schools. But since all models had at least a few individual sites which produced data suggesting the effectiveness of a particular model, the government viewed all models as having value. On this basis, all models were considered appropriate for dissemination. Perhaps even more surprising was the fact that the model which produced the best outcome (read Direct Instruction) received less funding during subsequent funding cycles. The rationale was that since Direct Instruction had already demonstrated its validity, it did not need as much money. It was further argued that those models with poor data would be validated if only they had more money. (Not surprisingly, none of these "wanna-be-valid" programs ever reached this criterion.) Clearly, neither data nor reason were relevant to these institutional actions. [1]

The Lesson

The moral of Follow Through and similar stories is that "having" the data, by itself, is not likely to change behavior at the institutional or individual level. Obviously, we need data to validate and refine our clinical practices. We need data to ensure that we are proceeding ethically. We may also need data to help apply contingencies in ways discussed later in this commentary. But having the data, by itself, may be akin to "talk therapy" with a reluctant client. Behavior analysts must discriminate the difference between talking about the data vs. applying contingencies to get others to behave in ways that are consistent with the data. We would not seek to change the behavior of a client by showing reprints from JEAB or JABA. Instead, we change the contingencies relevant to the target behavior. And so it should be with the individuals and institutions that request, fund, and install treatment practices for children with autism.

Potential Interventions

Intensive early intervention programs for children with autism, while expensive, are clearly cost-effective. The lifetime financial costs associated with caring for an individual with autism are in excess of $1,000,000. The cost of intensive early intervention for 3 years has been estimated to range from $99,000 - $150,000 (Jacobson, Mulick, & Green, in press).

While intensive behavioral intervention with young children is not expected to produce an independent "typical" adult in every case, the percentage expected to reach these goals, or make significant gains, makes intensive intervention for every child with autism a plan that will, over the long term, yield real savings. However, there are contingencies that interfere with this potential outcome from altering current behavior.

For example, it is the federal and state governments, in particular those associated with developmental disabilities (e.g., Departments of Developmental Disabilities), which realize savings from intensive early intervention. However, the public schools most frequently pay the cost of these treatments. From the public school's financial perspective, intensive early intervention will never be cost effective, even if every child achieved normal functioning. Other barriers include the fact that administrators' behaviors are consequated based on this year's fiscal budget, and not costs avoided in future funding cycles. Targeting these defective contingencies should increase the institutional dollars and interest for intensive behavioral intervention for children with autism.

Case law involving psychotherapy may also prove instructive. As Green (this volume) notes, recovered memory syndrome, a therapeutic practice that lacks experimental support, has resulted in substantial monetary damages being awarded to those harmed by its application. In addition, there are a few cases where therapists have been successfully sued by clients for failing to use the most efficacious treatment, as generally shown in the research, for a particular disorder. When the associated response costs (monetary awards) are high enough, such cases encourage therapists to utilize practices which have scientific merit. The field of autism could benefit from lawsuits which are similarly on point. Therefore, unlike Shakespeare's Dick in Henry VI, instead of "killing all the lawyers" we need to cultivate attorneys sympathetic to children and science. In order to achieve this, we need the data, and then we need to turn it over to those who know how to leverage it as part of a contingency.

Similarly, behavior analysis must find ways to support parents (perhaps on a pro-bono basis) who want behavioral intervention for their children. Some school districts will provide intensive behavior intervention programs for children with autism, not because they find the outcome data compelling, but because their school boards wish to avoid the time and money associated with due process complaints.

In addition, to the extent that professional reinforcers (such as recognition and deference) are strictly associated with academic endeavors such as research, there may be little motivation for behavior analysts to develop procedures that "sell" scientifically validated behavioral practices to the general public. We need to extrapolate from the concept underlying ABA's awards for those who effectively disseminate and represent behavior analysis in the media and to the general public. Clearly, we must do more to encourage such behaviors through explicit reinforcement contingencies.

As Skinner himself noted in his ABA address "Why We So Happy Few?", simply having the data and the methodology to address important social problems is not sufficient to guarantee implementation or even attract interest. We have built the field of behavior analysis. But "they" have not come. Fortunately, we have the analytic framework to change this state of affairs and therefore influence the fate of children with autism yet to be born.

Endnote

1. Attempts to understand these bizarre actions has been discussed in terms of self-serving contingencies affecting the behavior of various stakeholders including educational publishing companies, teacher training institutions, and school personnel. See Watkins (1988) for a discussion of the history of Project Follow Through and related educational malpractice.

References

Jacobson, J.W., Mulick, J.A., & Green, G. (in press). *Cost benefit estimates for early intensive behavioral intervention for young children with autism- General model and single state case*. Behavioral Interventions.

Watkins, C.L. (1988) Project Follow Through: A story of the identification and neglect of effective instruction. *Youth Policy, 10*, 9-11.

Chapter 2

The Behavior Interference Theory of Autistic Behavior in Young Children

Sidney W. Bijou and Patrick M. Ghezzi
University of Nevada, Reno

There are at least three behavioral theories of autism in young children: the behavioral hypothesis of Ferster (1961), the behavioral theory of Lovaas and Smith (1989), and the social communication theory of Koegel, Valdez-Menchaca and Koegel (1994). All are in agreement that young children with autism can be analyzed in terms of behavioral analytic concepts and principles, and that the same concepts and principles can be applied in the analysis and treatment of this disorder. They differ, however, on the on the immediate cause of autism. The Ferster hypothesis attributes autism to faulty parenting; the Lovaas and Smith theory to a mismatch between the nervous system of the child and the normal environment; and the Koegel, Valdez-Menchaca, and Koegel theory to a defective neurological or physiological process which can result in inappropriate socialization, and in turn to maladjustive behavior such as self-stimulation, defective language development, and tantrums. The Ferster hypothesis is supported by neither research nor clinical findings (Rimland, 1964, 1996); the Lovaas and Smith, and the Koegel, Valdez-Menchaca, and Koegel theories are reductionistic (Peele, 1981) in that they attribute the immediate cause to a vaguely defined biophysiological factor or process.

Although the behavior interference theory (Bijou & Ghezzi, 1996) is in the tradition of these theories, it does not attribute the immediate cause of autistic behavior to the parents, to a mismatch between the child's nervous system and the normal environment, or to a vaguely defined malfunctioning biophysiological process. In other words, it remains in the domain of the behavioral approaches that focus on the mutual and reciprocal interactions between an individual's behavior and the events and circumstances in the environment (Bijou, 1998: Kantor, 1959: Skinner, 1953, 1974).

The first point about the behavior interference theory is that it views autism as a developmental psychopathological disorder (Achenbach, 1988; Harris, 1989; LeBlanc, Schroeder, & Mayo, 1997; Lock, Banken, & Mahone, 1994; Rogers & Pennington, 1991; Sigman, 1989), one in which its characteristics change over the life span. In the first developmental phase, namely the infancy and early childhood period, the child with autism deviates from the normal child in that there is an impairment of social interactions including verbal and non-verbal communication, a restricted repertoire of activities, resistance to change, high degree of stereotypic behavior, and disturbed sensory functioning (Eisenberg & Kanner, 1956; Kanner, 1943). All of these characteristics vary on a continuum from low to high.

The second point is that the behavior interference theory attempts to relate the foregoing characteristics to their antecendent and prevailing conditions by postulating that: (a) Young children with autistic behavior have abnormalities in their sensory equipment, among them the tendency to escape from and to avoid tactile and mild auditory stimuli. These abnormalities are on a continuum with the normal functioning of these sensory modalities: they are on the negative side of the distributions. (b) This tendency forecloses, completely or partially, the possibility of a child developing conditional positive social stimuli which acquire reinforcing, discriminative, and generalized reinforcing functions during child caring activities. These functions are an essential part of the social-emotional bonds, generally referred to as attachment, that develop between the mother and her child. (d) Abnormalities of attachment lead to abnormalities in the future development of social, emotional, and verbal behavior, and the behaviors related to them, such as cognition behavior and symbolic play (Skinner, 1957). (e) The stereotypic behavior seen in many children with autism is on a continuum of exploratory behavior in normally developing infants and young children. In the early stages of development, stereotypic behavior in both normal and autistic young children serves to acquaint them with the physical environment. In the later stages, its continuation in children with autism serves a compensatory function for their lack of adequate social and verbal behavior. (f) The behavior characteristics of infants and young children with autism are interrelated on the basis of the deficits and behavioral characteristics that typify these children.

Tendency to Escape and Avoid Tactile and Auditory Stimuli

One of the characteristics of many young children with autism is their frequently disturbed sensory reactions: vestibular, tactile, proprioceptive, interceptive, auditory, olfactory, and vision systems. Such aberrations distort their development and are at the root of most of their behavioral characteristics. We shall focus here only on their aberrant reactions to tactile and auditory stimuli because it is these sensory modalities, particularly the tactile, that have powerful roles in the development of social-emotional and verbal development.

That children with autism tend to escape and avoid tactile stimuli is apparent from the fact that they are indifferent or resistive to cuddling, affectionate overtures, physical contact, eye-contact, and social interactions of every sort (Ornitz Ritvo, 1886: Wing, 1996). For example, reports of parents read like this: "He seemed unresponsive to his parents and did not raise his arms in anticipation of being picked up . . . " (Wing, 1996, p. 48). "He never showed an anticipatory response to being picked up; he seemed to look through people, stiffened when held, and ignored affection" (Ornitz & Ritvo, 1968, p. 168). "She failed to cry, to be held or fed, from birth on, and by six months of age, it became apparent that she did not smile at others. During the first and second years, she never indicated she wanted to be held by the mother" (Ornitz & Ritvo, 1968, p. 167).

Grandin (1992), who claims to be a "recovered" autistic person, recalled that, "My early reaction to touching was like a wild animal. At first, touching was aversive then it became pleasant . . . When people hugged me, I stiffened and pulled away to avoid the all-engulfing tidal wave of stimulation. The stiffening and flinching was like a wild animal pulling away" (pp. 108, 118).

Escaping and avoiding tactile stimuli are deemed to be a critical factor in the diagnosis of autism according to the American Psychiatric Association's Diagnostic and Statistical Manual of Mental Disorders (1994) " . . . in infancy there may be a failure to cuddle, an indifference or an aversion to affection or physical contact and that parents report that they have been worried about the child since birth or shortly afterwards because of the child's lack of interest in social interaction" (pp. 68-69).

Parents of children with autism also report that early on their children showed unusual reactions to auditory stimuli. "He may dislike certain sounds, but at the same time he is unresponsive to sounds in general so that people will wonder if he is deaf" (Wing, 1966, p. 7). "From three months, he was panicked by any loud noise and startled repeatedly if one moved suddenly near him. The sensitivity to loud noises persisted until he was 6 years old" (Ornitz & Ritvo, 1968, p. 169). And a child research psychiatrist concluded, "Auditory avoidance is common, particularly to loud noises and speech. The child moves away or covers his ears or becomes distressed" (Wing, 1966, p. 8).

Grandin (1995) recalled that, "When I was little, loud noise was also a problem, often feeling like a dentist's drill hitting a nerve. They usually caused pain . . . Minor noises that most people can tune out drove me to distraction" (p.67).

Further evidence that auditory stimuli are aversive to many children with autism is gleaned from a survey by Rimland and Edelson (1995) on parents' descriptions of their autistic child's behavior. In their review of 17,000 questionnaires, they found that approximately 40% of autistic children were reported to be unusually sensitive to sounds. And a correlational-questionaire study by Tomchek (1997) on 100 children with autism between ages 2.6 and 6.6 years concluded to be auditorily sensitive to loud noise and to be distracted by noise" (p.22).

Effect of the Tendency to Escape and Avoid Tactile and Auditory Stimuli

The tendency of children with autism to escape and avoid tactile and auditory stimuli has several ramifications including interfering with the initial development of conditional positive social stimuli which take on reinforcing, discriminative, and generalized reinforcing functions. Let us elaborate.

In the context of normal child-rearing activities, conditional social positive reinforcers evolve in normally developing infants in the following way (Bijou & Baer, 1965; Gewirtz, 1961; Wahler, 1967): As a mother engages in nursing, bathing, dressing and undressing her infant in bed, and so on, she naturally touches, hold, talks, and sings during these activities. Stimuli from the mother—her presence, proximity, odor, movements, holding, talking, and touching—acquire conditional social properties by virtue of their association with the presentation of positive unconditional stimuli (e.g., providing milk when hungry) and the removal of aversive stimuli (e.g., pulling down the window shade to remove the glare of the sun on the child's face) inherent in these activities. These conditional social stimuli begin to acquire a reinforcing function because they occur consequent to the infant's behavior. They also acquire a discriminative function since they will soon serve as signals that the caretaker is present and will probably provide the infant with positive unconditional stimuli, or will remove an aversive stimulus. Further, certain stimuli from the caretaker, notably her attention, approval, and disapproval which will occur in more than one deprivational state will acquire generalized reinforcing functions, i. e., they will have reinforcing effectiveness independent of a specific setting factor.

In the same context, conditional social positive stimuli and their subsequent functions will not develop, or will develop only partially, with infants with autism because of their tendency to escape and avoid the mother's tactile and auditory stumuli. In fact, the mother's mere presence will soon acquire conditional aversive properties since she will be associated with tactile and auditory stimuli that are aversive to the infant. Instead of anticipating the mother's presence by raising his or her arms, the infant tends to look away, and if able, moves away.

And between routine child-caring activities when a mother plays with her normally developing infant by cuddling, rocking, talking, singing, and so on, the tactile and auditory stimuli she provides are paired with the infant's joyful and active participation. But with an infant who has a tendency to escape and avoid tactile and auditory stimuli, the stimuli from the mother's playful activities are associated with the infant's' pulling away, covering the ears, and "gaze aversion" (Miranda, Donnelly, & Yonder, 1983). Hence, there is little or no chance that the mother's playful behaviors during the times between child-caring activities will acquire conditional social positive stimulus functions. If or when the autistic infant's resistance or unresponsiveness discourages the mother's affectionate and playful activities, the infant's resistance or unresponsiveness will be further strengthened by negative reinforcement.

Thus, an infant's and young child's tendency to escape and avoid tactile and auditory stimuli interferes with his or her development of conditional positive social stimuli and their subsequent acquisition of reinforcing, discriminative, and generalized reinforcing functions. These stimulus functions play a significant role in the development of attachment. In one of Lovaas' early publications (1966), he offered a similar analysis:

> Normal development presupposes the acquisition of a large variety of secondary reinforcers. It follows that the child who has failed to acquire such reinforcers, should demonstrate a deficiency in the behaviors which would have been reinforced. In the extreme case of complete failure to acquire secondary reinforcers, the child should evidence little, if any, social behaviors. That is, the child should fail to attend to people, fail to smile, fail to seek company, to talk, etc. because his environment has not provided him with the rewarding consequences for such behavior or because he is unable to appreciate that consequences are rewarding. It is apparent that

such failure in the acquisition of secondary reinforcers need not be complete, but may be partial. (pp. 118-119)

Attachment

Attachment, a metaphor for the close social-emotional ties that develop between a mother and her normally developing infant, evolves in phases, according to Bowlby (1969) and others (e.g., Siegel, 1996). In the first few months, the child differentiates between the principal caretaker and others, and directs more attention to the principal caretaker. For example, an infant begins to show a strong preference for being held or played with by the principal caretaker, and displays a wariness of others. During the next phase, from about 9 to 18 months, an infant' attention to a caretaker is heightened and he or she shows distress in the absence of the principal caretaker and greater comfort in his or her presence. For example, the infant may cry when left alone in a room with a stranger, and when in a room with the mother and a stranger, he or she will play near the mother and will look back or call her whenever the stranger makes an attempt at play. Wariness of strangers will ordinarily peak at about 13 months of age. In the final phase of infancy, around 18 to 24 months, the infant can tolerate separation from the pricipal cartaker for increasing lentghs of time and is comfortable with strangers.

This sequence can be entirely absent, partially absent, or delayed in an infant with autism (Rutter, 1978). The infant tends to ignore the caretaker or turns away in response to positive social overtures, rather than show a preference for being picked up, held, or played with. In some cases an infant may respond positively to the appearance of the caregiver, but show a noticeable lack of snuggling, eye-contact, and expressions of joyful comfort.

Several explanations have been given for the abnormalities of attachment in an infant with autism. According to Bowlby's ethnological-adaption theory (1969, 1973), they are due to a defect in the infant's inherited behavior-motivational system which regulates the behavior that maintains proximity to and contact with a discriminated, protective person, usually the mother, and all aspects of attachment behavior, from its initial activation to its actual production.

The cognitive view (e.g., Rogers, Ozonoff, & Masin-Cole, 1993) of the distortion of attachment in the infant with autism is that it is due to the infant's inability to construct a working model of self and parents, a position not unlike Leslie's (1989), which holds that the infant with autism has a deficit in the ability to represent things and events mentally.

Our position is that abnormalities in attachment are due to the absence or only partial development of conditional positive social stimuli. As we pointed out earlier, child-caring activities inherently include the mother's presentation of unconditional stimuli and the withdrawal of aversive stimuli. In a normally developing child, these are paired with social stimuli from the mother, and through the conditioning that naturally takes place in child-caring activities, they acquire conditional social positive properties. These conditional social stimuli soon acquire reinforcing, discriminative, and generalized reinforcing functions by virtue of the interactions between the mother and child. Through these processes, the caretaker becomes a powerful person in the infant's life, showing joy and security when she is near and discomfort and insecurity when she is absent.

Stereotypic Behavior

Stereotypic behavior, such as hand flapping, body rocking, and surface rubbing, seen in many children with autism poses a problem for psychologists. Frith (1993), for example, states: "We have as yet little idea what to make of the single-minded, often obsessive, pursuit of certain activities. With the autistic person, it is as if a powerful integrating force—the effort to seek meaning—is missing" (p. 114). Behavioral psychologists treat stereotypic behavior variously. Some consider it inconsequential. Foxx and Azrin (1973), for example, consider it as behavior "that has no apparent functional effect on the environment" and O'Brien (1981) added "which usually does not cause physical self-injury." Schriebman, Koegel, Charlop, and Egel (1990) describe it as " . . . stereotyped, repetitive movements, which seem to do nothing other than to provide sensory input for the child . . . " (p.765). Other behavioral psychologists treat stereotypic behavior as behavior motivated by a state of arousal (e.g., Kinsburne, 1980). In hypoarousal, the child is thought to need an optimal level of stimulation, and if it is not available, he or she engages in stereotypic behavior as a means of gaining sensory stimulation. In hyperarousal, on the other hand, the child is thought to be exposed to too much stimulation and therefore tends to engage in stereotypic behavior in order to reduce the arousal level. Still other behavioral psychologists (e.g., Lovaas, Newsom, & Hickman, 1987) view this behavior as operant behavior reinforced by "perceptual" stimuli (a combinaation of exteroceptive and interceptive stumuli). Contingent "perceptual" stimuli are posited because "afferent stimulation during repetitve movement comes from multiple receptors and is relatively complex and patterned" (Dickinson, 1974).

Our position is that stereotypic behavior is operant behavior which is an extreme variation of the normal exploratory behavior (Bijou, 1980) seen in infants and young children soon after they have acquired the necessary manual and motor abilities. For normally developing young children, exploratory behavior results in a repertoire of knowledge about the characteristics of objects, such as their hardness and softness properties, and what they can do to a person or others, as well as what a person can do to them (Kantor & Smith, 1975). In children with autism as well as those with severe retardation, exploratory behavior also yields, in the initial stage of development, a repertoire of knowledge about the physical world, but in the later stages of development, sterotypic behavior serves as compensation for their lack of adequate social and verbal abilities. That is to say, such children respond with stereotypic behavior to escape and avoid stiuations requiring social and verbal abilities (Durand & Carr (1987). Furthermore, studies have shown that stereotypic behavior in children with autism can be reduced by increasing the child's ability to engage in appropriate play (e.g., Epstein, Doke, Sajwaj, Sorrell, & Rimmer, 1974), in social behavior (Lovaas & Newsom, 1976), and in communication (verbal) behavior.

Analyzing stereotypic behavior as a class of operant behavior requires comment about its antecedent and consequent stimuli. There is little doubt that antecedent stimuli for exploratory behavior is any temporal, spatial, or movement properties of objects, including the physical aspect of the infant's body and the bodies of others (Bijou, 1980). However, there is some question about the contingent stimuli. As noted above, Lovaas, Newsom, and Hickman (1987) posit "perceptual stimuli" because they come "from multiple receptors and are relatively complex and patterned." In our view, there is no need postulate contingent "perceptual stimuli" since there is evidence that the contingent stimuli for stereotypic behavior are automatically generated by the response itself (Baumeister & Forehand, 1983; Skinner, 1957; Sundberg, Michael, Partington, & Sundberg, 1996; Vaughn & Michael, 1982). Skinner (1953) pointed out that:

> Some forms of stimulation are positively reinforcing although they do not appear to elicit behavior having biological significance. A baby is reinforced, not only by food, but by the tinkle of a bell or the sparkle of a bright object. Behavior which is consistently followed by such stimulation shows an increased probability. It is difficult, if not impossible, to trace reinforcing effects to a history of conditioning. (p. 83)

Originally, stereotypic behavior in a child with autism is weak, but becomes strong as evidenced by the fact that a disruption can generate protests, tantrums, and aggression. Part of the added strength results from inadvertent reinforcement by caretakers who "give in" because for them such behaviors are extremely aversive (Ferster, 1961). Repetition of this practice makes these behaviors the child's dominate way of responding to frustration, thereby creating some of the disagreeable behavior often associated with these children.

Interrelationships Among Traits and Abilities

Profiles of deficits, such as the inability to imitate, to show anticipatory reaching, to be aware of others, to respond to symbols, to participate in pretend play, to engage in social referencing, and to participate in social play, have been reported as typical of children with autism (see Siegel, 1996). They have also been reported to have many behavioral traits, such as seeking physical comfort, and hand-leading a person to indicate wants and needs. These behavioral deficits and characteristics have been viewed as symptoms of a defect in some biophysiological condition or process (e.g., Hobson, 1989), or in some hypothetical mental structure (e.g., Frith, 1989), or as isolated traits (Ferster, 1961; Lovaas & Smith, 1989). Another possibility is that they may be interrelated on the basis of inadequate social–emotional behavioral repertoires (e.g., Koegel, Koegel, Hurley & Frea, 1992; Koegel, Valdez-Menchaca & Koegel, 1994). In other words, without the initial development of conditional social positive stimuli in the initial stage of child-caring activities, there can be only limited development of later social and verbal behavior, and little or no normal development of cognitive, imaginative, symbolic, and other behaviors that are dependent on or related to verbal behavior. In sum, most of the abnormal behaviors of children with autism serve to compensate for their deficiencies in social-emotional and verbal behavior.

A number of studies on children with autism have focused on their atavisms—tantrums, self-injurious behavior, protests, whining, shrieking, screaming, aggression, non-compliance, and oppositional behavior. These are, in the main, socially reinforced operant behaviors that occur in normally developing children as well as children with other handicapping conditions. From this point of view, they should be considered as behaviors that can accompany autism (Koegel, Valdez-Menchaca, & Koegel, 1994)

Summary

The behavior interference theory is the first part of a developmental psychopathological theory of autism which postulates that a young child with autism has a tendency to escape and avoid tactile and auditory stimuli. This tendency interferes with the initial development of conditional positive social stimuli, which comes from the pairing of parental social stimuli with the unconditional positive stimuli and the removal of aversive stimuli that are inherent in normal child-rearing activities. In subsequent interactions with the mother, these conditional social stimuli acquire reinforcing, discriminative, and generalized reinforcing functions, and thereby create a strong social-emotional relationship between the mother and her child, referred to as attachment. Hence, the tendency of an infant and young child with autism to escape and avoid tactile and auditory stimuli results in abnormalities in attachment, which in turn results in disturbances in the future development of social-emotional and verbal behavior. Other features of the theory include: (a) An analysis of stereotypic behavior as a class of automatically reinforced operant behavior with two functions for a child with autism. In the early stages of development, stereotypic behavior serves to acquaint him or her with the ecological environment, as it does with a normally developing child, but in the later stages, it serves the child with autism with a compensatory function for his or here lack of social and verbal repertoires. (b) The behavioral characteristics of an infant and young child with autism are interrelated, centering on his or her deficits in social-emotional and verbal behavior.

References

Achenback, T.M. (1988). Developmental psychopathology. In M. H. Borsstein & M. E. Lamb (Eds.), *Developmental psychology: An advanced textbook* (2nd. ed., pp. 549-591). Hillsdale, NJ: Lawrence Erlbaum Associates, Publisher.

American Psychiatric Association (1994). *Diagnostic and statistical manual of mental disorders* (4th ed. , pp. 66-69). Washington, DC.

Baumeister, A. A. & Forehand, R. (1983) Stereotyped acts. In N. R. Ellis (Ed.), *International review of research in mental retardation, 6*, 55-96. New York: Academic Press.

Bijou, S. W. (1998). Empirical behaviorism. In W. O'Donohue & R. F. Kitchener (Eds.), *Handbook of behaviorism* (pp. 179-183). New York: Plenum Press.

Bijou, S. W. (1880). Exploratory behavior in infants and animals: A behavior analysis. *The Psychological Record. 30,* 488-495.

Bijou, S.W. & Baer, D. M. (1965). *Child development II: Universal stage of infancy.* Englewood Cliffs, NJ: Prentice Hall.

Bijou, S. W. & Ghezzi, P. M. (1996). Theories of autistic behavior in young children. Paper presented at the 22nd Annual Convention of the Association of Behavior Analysis, San Francisco, CA.

Bowlby, J. (1969). *Attachment and loss: Vol. 1 Attachment.* New York; Basic Books,

Bowlby, J. (1973). *Attachment and loss: Vol. 2 Separation.* New York; Basic Books.

Dickinson, J. (1974). *Proprioceptive control of human movement.* Princeton, NJ: Princeton Book Co.

Durand, V. M. & Carr, E. G. (1987). Social influence on "self-stimulatory" behavior. Analysis of treatment application. *Journal of Applied Behavior Analysis, 20,* 119-132.

Eisenbeg, L. & Kanner, L. (1956). Early infantile autism, 1943-1955. *American Journal of Orthopsychiatry, 26,* 556-566.

Epstein, L. H., Doke, L. A., Sajway, T., Sorrell, S., & Rimmer, B. (1974). Generality and side effects of over-correction. *Journal of Applied Behavior Analysis, 7.* 385-390.

Ferster, C. B. (1961). Positive reinforcement and the behavior deficits of autistic children. *Child Development, 32,* 437-456.

Foxx, R. M. & Azrin, N. H. (1973). The elimination of self-stimulatory behavior by over-correction. *Journal of Autism and Developmental Disabilities, 6.* 1-14.

Frith, U. (1989). *Autism: Explaining the enigma.* Oxford: Basel Blackwell.

Frith, U. (1993). Autism. *Scientific Monthly, 268,* 108-114.

Gewirtz, J. L. (1961). A learning analysis of the effects of normal stimulation, privation, and deprivation of the acquisition of social motivation and attachment. In B. M. Foss (Ed.) *Determiners of infant behavior* (pp. 213-299). New York: Wiley Publishing Co.

Grandin, T. (1992). An inside view of autism. In E. Schopler & G. E. Mesilov (Eds.), *High functioning individuals with autism* (pp. 105-126). New York: Plenum Press.

Grandin, T. (1995). *Thinking in pictures.* New York: Vintage Books.

Harris, P. L. (1989). The autistic child's impaired conception of mental states. *Journal of Autistic and Developmental Disorders, 11, 331-346.*

Hobson, R. P. (1989). Beyond cognition: A theory of autism. In G. Dawson (Ed.), *Autistism: New perspectives in diagnosis, nature and treatment* (pp. 22-48). New York: Guilford.

Kanner, L. (1943). Autistic disturbance of affective contact. *Nervous Child, 2,* 217-250.

Kantor, J. R. (1959). *Interbehavioral psychology* (2nd rev.). Bloomington, IN: Principia Press.

Kantor, J. R. & Smith, N. W. (1975). *The science of psychology: An interbehavioral survey.* Chicago: Principia Press.

Kinsbourne, M. (1980). Do repetitive movement patterns in children and animals serve a derousing function? *Journal of Developmental and Behavioral Pediatrics, 1,* 39-42.

Koegel, L. K., Koegel, R. L., Hurley, C. & Frea, W. D. (1992). Improving programmatic skills and disruptive behavior in children with autism through self-management. *Journal of Applied Behavior Analysis, 25,* 341-354.

Koegel, L. K., Valdez-Menchaca, M. C., & Koegel, R. L. (1994). Autism: Social communication difficulties and related behaviors. In V. B. Van Hasselt & M. Herson (Eds.), *Advanced abnormal psychology (pp. 165-187).* New York: Plenum Press.

LeBlanc, J. M., Schroeder, S. R., & Mayo, L. (1997). A life span approach in the education and treatment of persons with autism. In D. Cohen & F. R. Volkmar (Eds.) *Handbook of autism and pervasive developmental disorders* (2nd ed., pp. 1-24). New York: Wiley Publishing Co.

Leslie, A. M. (1989). Some implications of pretense for mechanisms underlying the child's theory of mind. In W. J. Astington, P. L. Harris, & D. R. Olson (Eds.), *Developing theories of the mind* (pp. 19-46). New York: Cambridge University Press.

Lock, B. J., Banken, J. A. & Mahone, C. H. (1994). The graying of autism: Etiology and prevalence at fifty. In J. L. Matson (Ed.), *Autism in children and adults* (pp. 37-57). Pacific Grove, CA: Brooks/Cole Publishing Co.

Lovaas, O. I. (1966). A program for the establishment of speech in psychotic children. In J. K. Wing (Ed.), *Early childhood autism: Clinical, educational and social aspects* (pp. 115-144). Oxford: Pergamon Press.

Lovaas, O. I. & Newsom, C.D. (1976). Behavior modification with psychotic children. In H. Leitenberg (Ed.), *Handbook of behavior modification and behavior therapy* (pp. 303-360). Englewood Cliffs, NJ: Prentice-Hall.

Lovaas, O. I., Newsom, C. D. & Hickman, C. (1987). Self-stimulatory behavior and perceptual reinforcement. *Journal of Applied Behavior Analysis, 20,* 45-68.

Lovaas, O. I., & Smith, T. (1989). A comprehensive behavior theory of autistic children: Paradigm for research and treatment. *Journal of Behavior Therapy and Experimental Psychiatry, 20,* 17-29.

Mirenda, P. L., Donnell, A. M., & Yoder, D. C. (1983). Gaze behavior: A new look at an old problem. *Journal of Autism and Developmental Disabilities. 13, 397-409.*

O'Brien, F. (1981). *Handbook of behavior modification with the mentally retarded.* New York: Plenum Press.

Ornitz, E. M. & Ritvo, E. R. (1986). Perceptual inconsistency in early infantile autism. *Archives of General Psychiatry, 18,* 76-98.

Peele, S. (1981). Reductionism in the psychology of the eighties. *American Psychologist, 86,* 807-818.

Rimland, B. (1994). The modern history of autism: A personal perspective. In J. L. Matson (Ed.), *Autism in children and adults* (pp. 1-11). Pacific Grove, CA: Brooks/Cole Publishing Co.

Rimland, B. & Edelson, S. M. (1995). Brief report: A pilot study of auditory integration training in autism. *Journal of Autism and Developmental Disabilities, 25,* 61-70.

Rogers S. J. Ozonoff, S., & Maslin-Cole, C. (1993). Developmental aspects of attachment behavior in young children with pervasive developmental disorders. *Journal of the American Academy of Child and Adolescent Psychiatry. 32,* 1274-1282.

Rogers, S. J. & Pennington, B. F. (1991). A theoretical approach to the deficits in infantile autism. *Development and Psychopathology, 3,* 137-162.

Rutter, M. (1978). Diagnosis and definition of childhood autism. *Journal of Autism and Childhood Schizophrenia, 8,* 139-161.

Schriebman, L., Koegel, R. L., Charlop, M. H. & Egel, A. L. (1990). Infantile autism. In A. S. Bellack, M. Hersen, & A. E. Kazdin (Eds.), *International handbook of behavior modification and therapy* (2nd ed., pp. 763-789). New York: Plenum Press.

Siegel, B. (1996). *The world of the autistic child.* New York: Oxford University Press.

Sigman, M. (1989). The application of developmental knowledge to a clinical problem: The study of childhood autism. In D. Cicchetti (Ed.) *Rochester symposium on developmental psychopathology, Vol. 1, The emergence of a discipline* (pp. 165-1787). Hillsdale, NJ: Erlbaum.

Skinner, B. F. (1953). *Science and human behavior.* New York: The Free Press.

Skinner, B. F. (1957). *Verbal behavior.* New York: Appleton-Century-Crofts.

Skinner, B. F. (1974). *About behaviorism.* New York: Alfred A. Knopf.

Sunberg, M. L., Michael, J. L., Partington, J. W., & Sunberg, C. A. (1996). The role of automatic reinforcement in early language acquisition. *The Analysis of Verbal Behavior, 13,* 21-37.

Tomchek, S. D. (1997). Sensory processing behavior in children diagnosed with autism spectrum disorder: An item analysis. *1997 ASA National Conference of Autism—Advocate pp.* 21-22.

Vaughan, M. E. & Michael, J. L. (1982). Automatic reinforcement: An important but ignored concept. *Behaviorism, 10,* 217-227.

Wahler, R. G. (1967). Infant social attachments: A reinforcement theory interpretation and investigation. *Child Development, 38,* 1079-1088.

Wing, J. K. (1966). Diagnosis, epidemiology and etiology. In J. K. Wing (Ed.), *Early childhood autism: Clinical, educational, and social aspects* (pp. 3-49). Oxford: Pergamon Press.

Acknowledgement

We thank our colleagues for reading the manuscript and offering valuable suggestions for the final revision. They include James E. Carr, Linda J. Hayes, Steven C. Hayes, and Robert F. Peterson.

Discussion of Bijou and Ghezzi

In Praise of Consistency of Premise:
A Reply to Bijou and Ghezzi

Linda J. Hayes
University of Nevada, Reno

Bijou and Ghezzi reject the theories of autism proposed by Lovaas and Smith (1989) and Koegel,Valdez-Menchaca and Koegel (1994) on the grounds that these theories, in attributing the immediate cause of autistic behavior to biological conditions, are reductionistic. Bijou and Ghezzi do not explain their objection to reductionism in this context. I assume, however, that their objection stems from the fact that reductionistic "solutions" to psychological problems merely locate these problems in the subject matter of another discipline which is as ill-prepared as the first to solve them at its own level of analysis, leading, inevitably, to further reduction. While getting rid of a problem in this way is a solution of sorts, it is not a solution to the problem at hand. It is a solution to a different problem – the problem of having to solve a problem. There is little value in this approach.

I suspect that it is not only the reductionism of these other theories that Bijou & Ghezzi find objectionable about them. It seems likely that they are also found wanting in empirical support, as was their rationale for rejecting Ferster's (1961) theory. Indeed, the biological circumstances to which autism is attributed in the theories of Lovaas et al and Koegel et al are hypothetical. The observed events giving rise to the term "autism" are psychological in nature. They consist of unusual patterns of responding with respect to stimulating – not mismatched nervous systems and defective neurological processes. Finally, the postulational background of the Bijou and Ghezzi theory suggests that the causal focus of these other theories might also be a point of contention. The Behavior Interference Theory is more field-theoretical than causal in formulation.

The Behavior Interefernce Theory of Bijou and Ghezzi shares some of these same problems, however. For example, like those of Lovaas et al and Koegel et al, the Behavior Interference Theory is reductionistic. Bijou and Ghezzi propose that autism may be traced to abnormalities of sensory equipment. Specifically, these authors suggest that sensitivity to environmental stimulation may be depicted as a continuum. Presumably, the low end of this continuum is evident in the facts of auditory and visual impairment, passing through a middle range in which most of us appear to operate, and proceeding to a high end of unusual sensitivity characteristic of persons with autism. A continuum of sensitivity to environmental stimulation is not an unreasonable suggestion. It is nonetheless still reductionistic to suggest that this sensitivity is an effect of biological causes, particularly when the biological circumstances held to play this role are hypothetical in kind. It is difficult for this author to appreciate the necessity of this formulation, given the more field-theoretical foundations upon which the Behavior Interference Theory is built beyond this rather unusual starting place.

The philosophical foundations of these various theories of autism, while worthy of consideration on their own terms, are perhaps not so important as their implications for the development of effective therapeutic practices. In this regard, I would argue that attributing psychological events to biological causes is an impediment to this development as it leaves in its wake a lingering doubt as to the possibility of a truly successful psychological intervention. In other words, if autism reflects biological abnormality, successful psychological interventions must be conceptualized as either being powerful enough to mask biological inadequacies or, alternatively, to correct them. The authors do not address this issue despite considerable evidence of successful psychological interventions with this population. Instead, Bijou and Ghezzi take abnormalities of biological equipment as a starting point from which abnormalities of psychological development proceed through a succession of organism-environment interactions. While their arguments concerning this development are exceptionally well formulated, the evidence of successful psychological interventions begs the question as to how the debilitating effects of abnormal biological development are overcome by these interventions.

Given no indication as to how such circumstances are overcome by psychological means, it seems plausible to surmise that no such circumstances are actually in place to begin with. That is to say, perhaps the assumption of abnormalities of sensory equipment as an initiating cause of autistic behavior is unnecessary. The alternative to this assumption is to suggest that psychological behavior of every variety, including sensory interaction, has ontogenic origins. From this perspective, what warrants speculation in the context of autism is how the development of sensory interactions might have been so unusual, and of such early onset, as to suggest biological abnormality. What follows is a suggestion in this vein.

As previously mentioned, Bijou and Ghezzi explicitly reject the faulty parenting hypothesis of Ferster (1961) on the grounds that it has not been substantiated by empirical findings. While I agree with their argument in this regard, speculation as to the nature of early sensory interactions of a sort that might eventuate in autistic behavior cannot avoid mention of parental involvement. In the absence of parental involvement, very young infants are able to interact with visual and tactile stimulation from relatively few sources. Auditory stimulation, likewise, is limited to ambient noise. It is, as such, only by way of parental actions that opportunities for interaction with a wider range of sensory stimulation become available to infants, particularly as they are moved from place to place so as to make contact with sources of such stimulation possible. Present speculations thereby depend on the incorporation of parental action in the analysis, although not as a causal matter of faulty parenting. The latter hypothesis is both unwarranted from the standpoint of a field-theoretical perspective in which causality is not isolated in a single factor but is rather interpreted as the organization of all participating factors (Kantor, 1959), as well as is unproductive of parental support in the implementation of corrective action. Moreover, evidence for the Ferster hypothesis is not pertinent to the present speculations, in that this evidence would be found, were it to be found, in interactions between parents and children at a latter point in their development than is the focus of these speculations. Hence, I will invoke different patterns of parental actions in the analyses to follow, although not in the role of causal variables for which blame may be assigned, and acknowledge that these analyses are not supported by empirical evidence.

If normal development of sensory interactions occurs by way of typical or usual opportunities for contact with sensory stimulation, then unusual patterns of contact with sensory stimuli may account for abnormal psychological development of this type. Parental actions figure prominently in very young infants' fields of sensory interaction, as previously mentioned. Such actions afford opportunities for contact with sensory stimulation that are otherwise unavailable to infants due to their limited ranges of independent motion. While affordances of these opportunities might be either more limited than is ordinarily the case, or available in the extreme, for purposes of illustration, we will consider only the latter case. First, however, we may consider the distribution of sensory interaction types typical of a normally developing infant and how this distribution changes over time. In making this analysis, I will be relying on the response deprivation hypothesis of Timberlake and Allison (1974.)

An infant's earliest psychological life is comprised of periods of highly varied sensory interaction afforded by parental care taking actions, periods of less varied stimulation when alone and relatively immobile, and periods of extremely little interaction of these sorts when asleep. As the infant matures, sleep periods decrease in both frequency and duration, while periods of more varied stimulation increase in both dimensions, this shift occurring as a function of both increasing independent mobility on the part of the infant, and increasing demands for parental involvement entailed in the care of an infant who is more often awake and for longer periods. The distribution of these patterns of sensory interaction continues to shift in this same direction over the course of normal development such that periods of highly varied sensory stimulation occupy an increasingly larger proportion of the infant's psychological life. It might be said that, as the infant matures, more varied sensory interactions come to be preferred over less varied interactions of this type, by way of which the former will be demanded. It is this development to which Bijou and Ghezzi refer in discussing the proclivity of normally developing infants toward exploratory behavior.

Because the very young infant is dependent on parental actions to afford opportunities for highly varied sensory stimulation, the distribution of periods of greater and lesser variability are largely determined by such actions. Returning, then, to the possibility of abnormal psychological development as a result of unusual patterns of contact with sensory stimulation, we may consider the circumstance in which periods of highly varied stimulation are elevated above preferred levels, and through which, periods of lesser variability are depressed below free operant baseline levels. In this case, participation in highly varied sensory stimulation afforded by parental interactions will become functionally aversive relative to the less varied stimulational circumstances afforded when the infant is alone.

If opportunities to participate in less varied stimulational circumstances were made contingent on participation in highly varied circumstances, that latter might be strengthened (Timberlake and Allison, 1974), in keeping with the preferences of the overindulgent parent. Competing with the arrangement of this contingency by the parent, however, is his or her preference for continuous interactions with the infant. That is to say, the periods of less varied stimulation permitted by the parent may be too brief and too infrequent to function effectively as reinforcement for participation in highly varied circumstances. The effect is to sustain the relative aversiveness of the highly varied circumstance, and to increase the likelihood of escape behavior on the part of the infant.

The infant has few means of effective escape, however. One means by which the infant is able to moderate the less than optimal distribution of stimulational types is to superimpose a less varied pattern of stimulation upon the highly varied pattern too often in place. Engaging in highly repetitive activity, through which visual and/or auditory stimulation from other sources may be partially blocked or minimized, may prove effective. Another potentially useful means of escape may be to shrink from tactile contact. These behaviors, should they occur, are likely to be sustained. Moreover, with repeated occurrences, these topographies are likely to become organized into more and more effective patterns, such that by the time the infant has reached the age of eighteen months or so they are able to be recognized and articulated as classic symptoms of early childhood autism.

The Behavior Interference Theory of Bijou and Ghezzi focuses on the development of these patterns after the fact of their presumed biological initiating conditions, along with their interactions with developing parental reactions to them. The Behavior Interference Theory is a particularly eloquent, field-theoretical description of these circumstances. The supposition of an initiating biological cause for this development, in this author's opinion, not only adds nothing of substance to this theory, but also draws into question the consistency of its philosophical foundation. One is led to wonder if the Behavior Interference Theory operates against a field-theoretical philosophical background or a causal one. If it were possible to construct a plausible sequence of strictly psychological interactions through which abnormal psychological development might take place, incorporating such an account into the Behavior Interference Theory would eliminate its apparent inconsistency.

References

Ferster, C. B. (1961). Positive reinforcement and the behavior deficits of autistic children. *Child Development, 32*, 437-456.

Kantor, J. R. (1959). *Interbehavioral Psychology*. Chicago: The Principia Press.

Koegel, L. K., Vladedez-Menchaca, M. C. and Koegel, R. L. (1984). Autism: Social communication difficulties and related behaviors. In V. B. Van Hasselt and M. Herson (Eds.) *Advanced Abnormal Psychology* (pp. 165-187). New York: Plenum.

Lovaas, O. I. and Smith, T. (1989). A comprehensive behavior theory of autistic children: Paradigm for research and treatment. *Journal of Behavior Therapy and Experimental Psychiatry, 20*, 17-29.

Timberlake, W. and Allison, J. (1974). Response deprivation: An empirical approach to instrumental perfromance. *Psychological Review, 81*, 146-164.

Chapter 3

Early Childhood Autism and Stimulus Control

Joseph E. Spradlin
Parsons Research Center
Nancy C. Brady
University of Minnesota

The term autism has been used in a variety of ways, however, it often refers to a particular set of behavioral limitations. Autism, as we understand it, refers to a subclass of pervasive developmental disorders (Mauk, Reber, & Batshaw, 1997). Children with autism are characterized as having impaired language, limited social interactions, and stereotyped behavior. A review of these limitations suggests that many impairments in social skills can be described in terms of limitations in the development of stimulus control. The advantage of this view of autism is that strategies that have proven effective in establishing new and complex stimulus relations may be applied prescriptively to the problems of autism. In this chapter, we will survey some of the specific problems that are exhibited by children with autism, then present hypotheses regarding the possible stimulus control limitations that could contribute to these problems. In addition, we will review some attempts to modify the stimulus relations associated with characteristic problems exhibited by children with autism.

Characteristics of Infants and Children with Autism

Social Skill Deficiencies

Deficiencies in social skills are perhaps the most common characteristics of children with autism (Volkmar, Carter, Grossman, & Klin, 1997). Parents give retrospective accounts that indicate that these deficiencies appear very early. Parents report that during the first months, infants with autism do not make normal eye contact (Mundy & Sigman, 1989) and do not seek physical contact with the parents (Kanner, 1943). Videos and films of children at their first birthday parties indicate that children who were later diagnosed as autistic showed less eye contact, imitated less, and were less likely to point out objects to others than were children who were later classified as normal (Osterling & Dawson, 1994). They may also fail to engage in simple reciprocal games such as pat-a-cake or peek-a-boo. They also exhibit less symbolic or make-believe play than do normally developing infants (Volkmar et al., 1997). There are also reports that children with autism are less likely to recognize emotional responses of other people (Volkmar et al., 1997).

Communication Skill Deficits

Closely related to problems in social behaviors are problems in language and communication. Children with autism are less likely to demonstrate multiple nonverbal communicative behavior such as joint attention (Mauk et al., 1997; Volkmar et al., 1997). That is, they are less likely to alternate between looking at an object and then looking at an adult's face as if to determine whether the adult was attending to the object. Joint attention paired with communicative gestures, such as pointing, are rare or absent in young children with autism (Baron-Cohen, 1989; Curcio, 1978; Mundy, Sigman, Ungerer, & Sherman, 1986; Wetherby, Yonclas, & Bryan, 1989). These behaviors exemplify early social communication in typically developing children. Children with autism are less likely to respond to their names and verbal directions than typically developing infants, and may appear deaf (Osterling & Dawson, 1994; Mauk et al., 1997). Their verbal behavior is more likely to be mands than tacts (Baron-Cohen, 1989; Ferster, 1961). Children with autism who develop speech are more likely to exhibit ecolalia and pronoun reversals than other children (Mauk et al., 1997) or they may use given names in place of pronouns (Lord & Rhea, 1997).

Stereotypies

Children with autism are more likely than normally developing children to engage in repetitive stereotyped behavior such as flicking their hands in front of their eyes or flipping a string, or twirling objects. There are also reports of them being very resistant to change, engaging in tantrums or self-injurious behavior when their routines have been modified in minor ways (Volkmar et al., 1997).

In spite of these reported extreme deficits, some children with autism are reported to exhibit normal or advanced skills in dealing with certain aspects of their nonsocial environment (Volkmar et al., 1997). For example, they may be able to put complex puzzles together or echo long jingles heard on television.

Thus far, we have described classic characteristics of children with autism. In the following section we will discuss these behaviors in terms of possible stimulus control limitations.

Stimulus Control Limitations: Implications for Autistic Behavior

In the following pages, we ask whether many of the characteristics of children with autism are not a function of stimulus control limitations. We ask whether stimulus control limitations ranging from the basic reflexive behavior of infants, to the complex stimulus control found in equivalence, would result in autistic characteristics. Throughout our discussion of possible limitations in stimulus control, we have a guiding hypothesis (perhaps wild speculation is the more appropriate term) that infants and children with autism require a greater consistency of stimulus, response, and reinforcement relations for stimulus control to develop than do typically developing infants and children. Moreover, we hypothesize that the contingencies involved in interacting with the nonsocial physical world are much more consistent than those involved in social interactions. Hence, infants with autism may be less controlled by social stimuli, and relatively more controlled by the nonsocial physical environment. The hypothesis that inconsistent social contingencies lead to the behavior deficits of children with autism is not new. Nor is the hypothesis new that the nonsocial environment provides a more consistent set of contingencies. Ferster (1961) proposed that intermittent reinforcement and extinction resulted in a loss of socially oriented behaviors, and that consistent nonsocial contingencies resulted in some of the stereotyped behaviors of children with autism. However, two aspects of our hypothesis differ from Ferster's. First, we focus on stimulus control limitations; Ferster mentioned stimulus control, but did not elaborate. Second, the implication of Ferster's hypothesis was that autism resulted from parenting failure. Our speculation is that children with autism differ from typically developing infants in the ease with which stimulus control is established. Hence, child rearing practices that are adequate for establishing stimulus control in typically developing infants and children are inadequate for establishing stimulus control in children with autism.

Primitive Stimulus Control and Reinforcing Stimuli

There may be differences in the reinforcing functions of various stimuli existing from birth. From birth environmental events control certain behaviors of typically developing infants. For example, typically developing newborn infants track objects such as faces (Brazelton, Koslowski, & Main, 1974). It seems possible that the visual patterns and movements of the human face constitute reinforcement for the orienting behavior of infants. Moreover, it has been suggested that certain types of physical contacts such as hugging or tickling are primary reinforcers (Charlop-Christy & Kelso, 1997). However, it has also been noted that some children with autism avoid such contact (cf. Bijou & Ghezzi present volume). Is it possible that some infants with autism differ from typically developing infants in the degree to which the sight of faces and the experience of hugging and tickling are reinforcers? If that were true, could that not result in social aloofness and being less interested in people?

Classical Conditioning Limitations

Some of the infants' earliest behaviors are reflexes; that is, they are unconditioned responses to unconditioned stimuli. For example, a touch to the cheek of a typical newborn infant elicits a rooting response, and a touch to the lip may elicit a sucking response. Papousek (1992) found that a neutral stimulus (a tone) paired with stimuli that elicited the rooting response could become a conditioned stimulus eliciting a rooting response. This conditioning process could account for the finding that some hungry breast-fed infants root in the direction of their mother's voice. It has also been noted that during the first weeks of life most infants become conditioned to footsteps, such that if they are whimpering or crying, they stop when the footsteps approach (Gekoski, Rovee-Collier, & Carulli-Rabinowitz, 1983). Similarly, many infants quiet when they hear a voice that has been paired with comforting (Thoman, Korner, & Beason-Williams, 1977). A question now arises: Do infants who will later be described as having autism also show such conditioning, or do such infants fail to develop such conditioned responses? For example, do they fail to become conditioned to footsteps or their mother's voice? The nonlaboratory world of infants is often inconsistent in its pairing of social stimuli with unconditioned stimuli. If infants with autism require more consistent pairings than other infants for conditioning to occur, they may be less likely to become conditioned to social stimuli and more likely to be conditioned to nonsocial aspects of their physical environment.

Limitations in Learning Simple Discriminations

While we speak of a discriminative stimulus as setting the occasion for a response to be reinforced, that does not imply that each time a response occurs in the presence of that stimulus that the response will be reinforced. Perhaps children with autism require that a higher percentage of responses in the presence of a stimulus be followed by the same consequence, if they are to come under the control of that stimulus. If this were true, it might explain once again why autistic children seem to prefer playing with objects rather than with people. The contingencies in the physical world may be more reliable than the contingencies of the social world. For example, when one sees an object close by and reaches out, he or she will almost inevitably be reinforced by certain tactile stimuli. Or when an infant sees a pacifier and places it in the mouth, the effect will be quite consistent from occasion to occasion. However, if a child makes a specific response in the presence of a parent or caretaker, the consequences may not be consistent from occasion to occasion. For example, if the child reaches for the parent, in a gesture to be picked up, on some occasions the child may be picked up, but on other occasions the parent may ignore the child's gesture. This lack of consistency may result in a child who does not come under the control of social stimuli.

Above, we noted the possibility that typically developing infants and infants with autism differ in the degree that certain stimuli are reinforcers at birth and noted that if tickling, cuddling, and affection were reinforcers at birth, children with autism might be less reinforced by these stimuli than were their typically developing peers. Bijou and Ghezzi (this volume) postulate that children with autism actually find physical contact aversive from birth. However, there are other possibilities. Perhaps hugs, tickles, and affection are initially neutral stimuli which become reinforcers because they are discriminative for reinforcers such as food, warmth, and diaper changes. If that is the case, possibly these stimuli fail to become conditioned reinforcers because children with autism require a much more consistent relation between primary reinforcers and stimuli for those stimuli to develop discriminative properties. Conditioned reinforcement largely depends on the stimulus being discriminative (Keller & Schoenfeld, 1950).

Numerous studies have demonstrated anomalies when children with autism were taught discriminations in one setting or context and then tested in slightly modified conditions. Perhaps the best known studies of anomalies in stimulus control are the studies of overselectivity. In these studies the child is reinforced for responses when multiple stimuli, such as bright light, white noise, and a tactile stimulus are presented simultaneously (Lovaas, Schreibman, Koegel, & Rehm, 1971). Researchers have found that children with autism often learn to respond to some of the stimuli, but not to all of the stimuli of the stimulus complex (Lovaas & Schreibman, 1971; Lovaas et al., 1971; Lovaas & Schreibman, 1979). For example, in the Lovaas et al. (1971) study, three children with autism responded primarily to the auditory stimulus and failed to respond to the visual and tactile stimuli, and two children with autism responded primarily to the visual stimulus and failed to respond to the auditory and tactile stimuli.

Sundberg & Partington (this volume) have argued that language training programs for children with autism will be most effective if they specifically teach echoic, tacts, and intraverbals. The classification of verbal behavior into echoics, tacts, and intraverbals is based on stimulus control. Typically developing children do not require independent teaching for these various kinds of stimulus control to develop. They develop even though, or perhaps because, most control of verbal behavior involves multiple stimulus control. For example, a child may be presented a toy truck accompanied by the verbal model "truck." The child may echo, "truck." Now, initially the typically developing child's response may be solely under the control of the verbal model; however, after one or more pairings the child may respond "truck" to the truck even when no model is present. Likewise the typically developing child may be asked "What hauls things?" and then given the model "truck." The child may soon be able to respond appropriately in the absence of the model. However, if a child is overselective, he or she will fail to respond to one of the stimuli in the setting. That is, when the child learns to say the word "truck" in response to a verbal model and the object truck, subsequently the child might respond consistently to the verbal model, but fail to respond when the truck is presented alone. A child who is overselective in such situations will be echolalic.

Limitations in Learning Conditional Discriminations

Much, perhaps most, conventional stimulus control is conditional. That is, a response to a stimulus is reinforced when a conditional stimulus is present, but not when the conditional stimulus is not present. For example, a request for play by a child may be honored by an adult when the adult is not otherwise engaged, but may not be honored if the adult is engaged in completing an income tax form or in a discussion with another adult. In a sense, a conditional discrimination involves a degree of inconsistency. That is, when a given discriminative stimulus is present a specific response will be reinforced only some of the time, namely when a conditional stimulus is present. Typically developing children seem to master easily such discriminations in their natural environment. Hence, they are reinforced for a high percentage of the responses they make in the presence of such discriminative stimuli. However, a child who fails to make that conditional discrimination will make many responses to the stimulus when the conditional stimulus is not present and may ultimately extinguish all responses to the discriminative stimulus. If a child fails to learn the subtle conditional discriminations involved in social behavior, social responding may be extinguished. Such limitations might be based on a more general failure to come under stimulus control unless the consequences for responding are highly consistent under a given stimulus condition. Our hypothesis is that such consistency is found relatively infrequently in the social world.

A particular example of conditional responding occurs when one shifts from being a listener to being a speaker. As a speaker, the people conventionally speak of themselves as I or me. However, as a listener, references to oneself become you. Likewise when one speaks to the second person one speaks to the person as you, but when that person speaks they will speak of the same referent as I. Perhaps a limitation in conditional discrimination leads a child with autism to speak of him or herself by the first name and his or her listener by a given name rather than by the pronouns you and I.

Limitations in Stimulus Class Acquisition

Much complex human behavior depends on the development of classes of stimuli that share no defining physical properties. For example, the spoken word "dog" and a picture of a dog do not share defining physical properties. Nevertheless, these stimuli are closely linked because of shared functions. If a new response or relation is established to one of these stimuli through training, then that response or relation may be established for the remaining stimulus without additional training. For example, if a child is taught to select the printed word DOG in response to the spoken word "dog," and a picture of a dog in response to the spoken word "dog," the child may also select the printed word DOG in response to the picture of the dog or the picture of the dog in response to the printed word DOG. Moreover, if the child is able to label the picture as "dog," he or she may also label the printed word as "dog" (Sidman, 1971). Or if the child develops an emotional response to a real dog, he or she may also exhibit that emotional response to the picture or spoken word "dog." There is evidence that some young children with autism are limited in their development of stimulus classes consisting of members without defining physical properties (Eikeseth & Smith, 1992). Now to what kinds of deficiencies might such limitations lead? There would be substantial deficits in language development. A child who did not develop equivalence classes might be quite able to echo speech; however, that speech might have no relation to the objects and events that are typically related to that speech. That is, the child's speech would not be meaningful. Such a child might also read, but not understand what was read.

Limitation in the Recombination of Minimal Stimulus-Response Units

Much human behavior involves responding appropriately to relatively novel situations. Two examples of such appropriate responding to novel situations are (a) imitation of a sequence of responses that one has never before imitated (generalized imitation), and (b) following a verbal instruction that one has never previously encountered. Let us consider generalized imitation first. Since generalized imitation occurs early in life, and for typically developing children without special tuition, it is easy to overlook what is involved in generalized imitation. For an observer not involved in the imitative act, the stimuli produced by the model and the imitator may appear quite similar. Early writers on imitation training actually spoke of similarity being a conditioned reinforcer (Baer, Peterson, & Sherman, 1967). But, if one looks at imitation from the point of view of the imitator, while there is a one-to-one correspondence between behavior exhibited by the model and the behavior of the imitator, there is little similarity between what the imitator sees and the specific stimuli produced by the imitator's own behavior (Siegel & Spradlin, 1978). In the imitation situation the relation between the behavior exhibited by the imitator and the stimuli exhibited by the model is every bit as dissimilar as are the spoken words of a person giving instructions and the behavior of the person who follows those instructions. We speculate that the development of generalized imitation occurs exactly as the development of instruction-following behavior. That is, by being taught to imitate multiple examples, the imitator learns a number of minimal stimulus response units, which then may be recombined when the imitator is presented a novel combination of responses for imitation. As noted in the section on the characteristics of children with autism, children with autism are often reported to have deficient imitation skills (Heimann, Ullstadiu, Dahlgren, & Gillberg, 1992; Stone et al., 1990). Rogers and Pennington (1991) view imitation as a social skill and stress that deficits in imitation could be devastating to the development of other social skills such as language. Children with autism in the Heimann et al. study did fairly well in imitating object manipulations, but performed poorly in imitations that did not involve objects.

As is the case for generalized imitation, typically developing children learn to follow relatively novel instructions at an early age. Most 2-year-old children follow basic three-word commands such as, "Pass the bread" (Miller, Chapman, Branston, & Reichle, 1980). Of course, such appropriate responding might be made simply on the basis of conditional discriminations. However, children who are able to respond by recombining units will be more effective, because if they have the appropriate word-object and word-action equivalencies, they can also respond to such combinations as "Butter your bread" and "Pass the salt." Moreover, if the child has learned certain equivalencies, and has learned the verbal responses to these equivalence classes, he or she will be able to make a variety of his or her own requests. However, these recombinations involve many conditional discriminations and a set of equivalence classes that may be quite limited in children with autism. What if a child were very limited in his or her ability to respond to recombinations of stimulus units? Such a child would be able to complete seemingly complex chains of behavior provided the chains were invariant. However, if a performance involved performing a series of responses on the basis of a novel instruction, they would fail.

Stimulus Control Issues and Theories of Mind

Recently Baron-Cohen and Swettingham (1997) summarized Baron-Cohen and colleagues' position that the problems of autism are symptomatic of an inadequate or lacking theory of mind. They note a variety of limitations indicating that children with autism are very poor at inferring what others are experiencing. In some ways, the general conception of a theory of mind or theories of minds has a kind of intuitive appeal. When one person speaks to another person, doesn't the speaker assume that the listener is hearing and understanding what the speaker is saying? We think such inferences about other peoples' minds are rather common when one person attempts to communicate with another person. Baron-Cohen and Swettingham list a variety of behaviors of children with autism that suggest that they aren't very good at inferring other peoples' experiences. For example, they are less likely to point out aspects of their environment to others, and they seem not to respond emotionally to others' joy or pain. They do not produce the same number of mental words as typically developing children, and they do not engage in as much pretend play.

At this point we are going to climb a long way out on a very small limb. Skinner (1957) made quite an issue of the role of private stimuli in human behavior. Now, the very definition of private stimuli precludes one person from ever experiencing another persons' private thoughts, emotions, or feelings. Yet, when most of us see another person experience an injury and turn white, wince, and cry, we almost automatically infer that that person is in pain. That is, we infer that that person is experiencing something similar to what we have experienced from a similar injury. In some cases we may almost feel the pain ourselves. If a small child points to an object and looks at us, we assume the child has seen something similar to what we are seeing. Each of us seems to make certain inferences concerning what other people are experiencing. In other words, we make inferences and these inferences might be called a theory of mind. Now, if typically developing children develop inferences about what other people are seeing, feeling, and thinking, how could this occur?

First, could *basic classical conditioning* play a role in the development of the inference that others experience private stimuli similar to our own? Consider the example of a child who bumps against the floor or the wall. The child may hear the bang of bumping the wall, experience pain, and cry. After a number of such experiences, the child may see another person bump the floor or wall and hear the bang of the wall being bumped. Could the child, as a function of the classical conditioning, be conditioned to cry in response to such an event? Or, consider a child who has been punished by scolding. The child may experience pain and cry. Now that same child may also come to cry when another child is scolded. And finally, it is possible that the mere sight of another child crying is sufficient to evoke similar emotional responses in some children. Is it possible that because of classical conditioning, these stimuli could elicit certain pain-like responses in the child? If so, is it also possible that certain limitations in classical conditioning among some children with autism could lead to a failure to develop appropriate emotional responses when another person is injured or showing the effects of such injury?

Second, could *generalized imitation* play a role in the development of a theory of mind? When a child imitates a model, the child not only is responding to the stimuli presented by the model, but also is responding to private kinesthetic and tactile stimuli. Is it possible, as the child becomes a proficient generalized imitator, that another person's behavior may evoke minimal implicit kinesthetic responses that were once related to imitating models? If so, the child might come to experience something similar to what the observed person is experiencing. Could a child who has learned to imitate proficiently infer that when the other person engages in a behavior that the person has the same private experiences as the child? We would speculate that a child who has a minimal or no imitative repertoire would be quite limited in the ability to make inferences concerning the private experiences of another person. Children with autism are often limited in their ability to imitate. Could this limitation result in a failure to develop a theory of mind?

Third, could *stimulus class development* play a role in the development of theories of mind? We speculate that stimulus classes play a major role in the development of theories of minds. This is especially true when some members of the stimulus class are conventional spoken or written words. When a person speaks, both the speaker and listener are subjected to auditory stimuli that are quite similar. Now the mere fact that two people are subject to that same auditory stimulus doesn't allow one to make the inference that their private experiences are similar. For example, when the model says "The block is red" and the child with autism echoes "The block is red," their basic experiences may be only minimally similar. For the model, the spoken words are representative. That is the word "block' is a unique member of an equivalence class that includes many different types of blocks and the printed word *block*. Similarly, the word "red" is a unique member of an equivalence class and the words "the" and 'is" combine to designate a particular type of relation. For the child with autism, perhaps the only relation involved is the relation between the spoken model and what is echoed. However, for typically developing members of a community, certain equivalencies will have been established in most members, such that they will share many equivalencies. Our hunch is that these shared observable equivalencies make it very likely that members will infer private events similar to those they experience when in a given situation. It would seem that children who do not develop conventional language would be quite limited in their theory of mind, since they would not share this wide range of conventional equivalencies.

The Use of Operant Teaching Methods with Children with Autism

As we have stated, children with autism seem to have considerable difficulty learning in an unstructured environment. Successful teaching programs have established stimulus control by structuring consistent relations between specified stimuli, behavior, and consequences. In the following paragraphs we will review several procedures for teaching children with autism to determine what aspects of the treatment were directed toward establishing new stimulus control by programming consistent stimulus-behavior-consequence relations. The procedures we have selected for review are drawn primarily from Charlop-Christy and Kelso's book "How to Treat the Child with Autism." However, many of the procedures are representative of the early stages of teaching for other programs, and may be traced to Lovaas' early work (Lovaas, 1977).

Procedures to Overcome Basic Reinforcer Problems

Charlop-Christy and Kelso suggest a number of procedures for overcoming reinforcement problems. They note that early in training, social events such as praise, smiles, and high fives may not be effective reinforcers, so they suggest the use of reinforcers such as foods or liquids, allowing the person to engage in stereo-typed behavior, or providing objects related to obsessions. In other words, they start by consistently presenting known reinforcers contingent on desired behaviors. They also suggest the use of token systems. Initially during training, to establish the token as a conditioned reinforcer, the token is given to the child and immediately ex-changed for a known reinforcer. That is, there is a consistent relation between the token and reinforcement. After this initial training the teacher may require that two tokens be received before they can be exchanged for a known reinforcer. Gradually, the number of tokens required prior to exchange is increased. Concurrently during training, praise is provided contingent on each desired response. No doubt the initial consistent delivery of tokens, praise, and a known reinforcer aids in establishing both the token and praise as reinforcers. One might ask why the token is presented. Why not simply start with establishing praise as a conditioned reinforcer? Our hunch is that such a procedure would be less effective, because it is difficult to maintain the same consistency in the relation of praise to known reinforcers as is possible with the token. Each token is like every other token. However, the intensity and quality of social events vary from occasion to occasion.

Basic Discrimination Training Procedures

When we reviewed specific training targets, we found that behavioral charac-teristics of children with autism were attacked directly, and that the procedures used often involved teaching new and conventional stimulus control. One of the first targets of the Charlop-Christy and Kelso (1997) program was the reduction of stereotyped behavior. The recommended procedure was to establish the verbal command "Hands flat" as a discriminative stimulus for placing the hands on the knees. While initially the child might need prompting to place his or her hands down, later the child is reinforced for longer periods of having his or her hands on his or her knees. So stereotyped behavior is reduced by establishing new behavior, initially under the control of a verbal instruction, and probably later under the control of the general training setting.

The next target for training is eye contact. According to Charlop-Christy and Kelso, and consistent with the definition, almost all children with autism lack this social skill. The basic procedure involves the teacher seated facing the child, having the child seated quietly, and the teacher saying, "Look at me." If the child makes even a fleeting glance, the child is reinforced with a tangible and praise. If the child does not look at the teacher, the teacher engages in one or more of the following prompts: the teacher places his or her finger right between his or her eyes while saying the child's name, or touches the child's chin and lifts his or her face to a position where the child can easily view the teacher's face. Whenever the child looks at the teacher, the child is reinforced. This procedure is repeated until the child is looking at the teacher on command for 8 of 10 trials. The prompts for looking at the teacher's face are gradually faded. This procedure seems ideal, not only for directly increasing an important behavior (eye contact), but also for developing a person's eyes and face as a conditioned reinforcer.

Early Childhood Autism and Stimulus Control

Establishing New Forms of Conditional Stimulus Control

One of Charlop-Christy and Kelso's early targets of training is compliance. The procedures for compliance training start with getting the child's attention by saying "Look at me" or "Pay attention," then giving a simple directive. The directive may be a verbal request such as "Sit down" or a request to imitate. For example, the teacher may obtain the child's attention, say, "Do this" and then provide a model such as clapping the hands. If the child claps his or her hands, the child is reinforced with both a tangible and social descriptive praise. If not, the teacher may manually guide the response and then provide reinforcement. The model is then presented again; if the child responds correctly, he or she is reinforced, if not he or she may be manually guided again. Another example of conditional discrimination training involves teaching receptive labels. Several objects may be placed in front of the child and the child is reinforced when the object requested by the teacher is selected. On different trials the teacher will request different objects.

Teaching Stimulus Classes

Forming conditional discriminations is a basis for the development of equivalence classes. While the Charlop-Christy and Kelso program does not specifically test to determine whether equivalence classes have been formed, many of their techniques would seem to promote such classes. For example, in preparing a child for picture communication, they teach the child to match pictures to objects. They also teach the child to select pictures in response to spoken words. Such a procedure may be sufficient to establish the picture, the object, and the spoken word as members of an equivalence class. The likelihood that the picture, object, and spoken word become members of a common equivalence class is made more likely because they encourage the child to echo the spoken word. Making a common response to two different stimuli enhances the chances that they will become members of the same equivalence class (Eikeseth & Smith, 1992). Nevertheless, the program might be improved if tests were made to determine if the stimuli had become members of an equivalence class, because such training does not necessarily result in equivalence classes.

Teaching Recombination of Stimulus-Response Units

One of the earliest attempts to treat autistic children involved an attempt to establish imitative behavior (Metz, 1965). Initially, the children in Metz's study did not imitate. However, through a variety of prompting techniques and the systematic delivery of reinforcement contingent on behavior that matched the trainer's behavior, the children began to imitate specific trained behaviors. After being taught a certain number of imitative responses, the children were able to imitate responses for which they had not been specifically trained. As stated above, our hunch is that such imitation of novel responses depends on recombination of previously learned minimal units.

Charlop-Christy and Kelso (1997) recommend a similar procedure to teach a child with autism to follow directions. The child is given a simple direction. If the child complies, he or she is reinforced. If not, the teacher continues to ensure that the directive is followed. This may involve manual guidance. So the procedure is once again consistent: follow the directive and receive reinforcement, fail to follow the directive and be manually guided through. Once again the procedure would be ideal for a child who failed to learn under inconsistent contingencies. An example of compliance training suggests that their procedures involve a substantial amount of recombination of units. Three examples were "Give me," "Go get," and "Put on." Now, it is possible that these directives are simply learned as a single unit. However, if the child is given a variety of directives such as "Give me plane," "Go get paper," "Go get the coat," "Give me the coat," and "Put on coat," then the child may begin to respond to "Go get," "Give me," and "Put on," as units and "coat," "plane," and "paper" as units that can be recombined so that the child may later respond appropriately to directives involving new combinations of the units he has previously learned. While the program appears to provide training that could result in the child being able to respond to commands involving novel recombination of units, the program itself does not include specific tests for adequate performance of such commands. It might be well if directives for training were selected so that units were recombined during compliance training, and tests were made to determine if the child follows directives consisting of untrained combinations.

Compliance training can be viewed as the first step in establishing receptive language (listener behavior). The Charlop-Christy and Kelso (1997) program goes far beyond teaching appropriate responses to simple directives. It includes procedures for teaching the concepts of same and different, appropriate responses to prepositions, to temporal labels such as before and after or first and last, and sequential responses to verbal directives. If I understand the training procedures, all of these are attempts to establish conventional stimulus control, and all initially involve continuous immediate reinforcement for making a specific response, or set of responses, to a specific stimulus or set of stimuli.

Picture Communication as a Stimulus Control Example

Since approximately 50% of children with autism do not talk, and even those who do talk may not respond well to spoken directives, there have been recent attempts both to teach children with autism to communicate by picture selection techniques (Bondy & Frost, 1994) and to instruct students by the use of pictures (Krantz & McClannahan, in press; MacDuff, Krantz, & McClannahan, 1993).

Perhaps the most prevalent use of pictures with children with autism has been aimed at teaching them to request by pointing to pictures or by giving pictures to others. One such program, the Picture Exchange Communication System (Bondy & Frost, 1994) encourages student-initiated requests. The first step in the Picture Exchange Communication System (and many other programs) is to identify a number of foods, objects, or activities that are potential reinforcers for the child's behavior. The next step in the Picture Exchange Communication System is to teach the child to exchange a picture for one of the reinforcers. Communication partners are to wait until the child initiates, then begin teaching. For example, as the child reaches for a piece of candy, a trainer redirects the reach toward the picture of candy, assists the child in picking up the picture, and assists in releasing it to a communication partner. The partner then immediately provides the candy. Verbal prompts are forbidden during the initial stages of the picture exchange. Subsequent teaching steps increase the variety and length of communications (e.g., 2-word phrases are introduced by placing a picture of a reinforcer next to a symbol indicating "I want").

In terms of the hypotheses presented in this chapter, the Picture Exchange Communication System effectiveness may be due to the reliance on consistent environmental contingencies while minimizing spoken input. Verbal antecedents are typically variable and somewhat unpredictable. In addition to developing communication initiation, programs such as the Picture Exchange Communication System may result in the communication partners becoming conditioned reinforcers. The pictures should also become conditioned reinforcers because they are discriminative for reinforcement by the foods, objects, and activities pictured. The communication partners may become generalized conditioned reinforcers because they are discriminative for the delivery of a variety of reinforcers. The Picture Exchange Communication System also incorporates the re-combination of units in its teaching of simple sentence construction. Students are taught to combine "I want" with many different object pictures. Later, they are taught to combine "I see" with these same pictures.

While pictures can be used to aid children in requesting and naming, they have also been used to instruct children to carry out a sequence of activities. Krantz and her colleagues have used pictures to guide children with autism through a sequence of independent play activities (MacDuff et al., 1993). Basically, their procedure is to teach children with autism to be guided by a book consisting of a series of pictures representing specific play activities. After training is completed, children with autism are able to, after looking at a picture, go get the play materials pictured, play appropriately with the materials, return the materials to the appropriate place, then go back to the book and turn to the next picture and engage in the next play activity. They have been able to teach young children with autism to go through a series with as many as 15 play activities independently. Moreover, they have demonstrated that the pictures do control the sequence of activities by rearranging the sequence of pictures. The success demonstrated in controlling a long series of play behaviors through the use of pictures raises a number of issues. Perhaps it is not surprising that children can be taught a routine or chain of behaviors, involving looking at a picture, going and getting materials, playing with those materials, and replacing those materials. The sequence is no doubt very consistent, and the contingencies within the sequence consistent. Moreover, once trained, the activity does not involve the inconsistencies of the behavior of other people. The fact that the behavior is not disrupted when the pictures are rearranged is interesting, because it demonstrates, first, that the specific pictures are controlling the order in which the children engage in the various play activities, and also that the specific routines controlled by each picture can be recombined in different orders. Now, why is the picture procedure so effective in controlling behavior? Is it because the picture is a permanent stimulus in contrast to spoken or gesture commands, which are transitory? Is it because the picture is always the same, while spoken or gesture directives vary from trial to trial? Or is it because the picture is somewhat iconic with the play activity? Would the same results be obtained with arbitrary symbols as with the pictures? In other words, are the pictures representational?

Stimulus Control Procedures to Develop Theories of Mind

Behavior analysts have understandably not focused on teaching theories of mind. Nevertheless, we speculate that certain skills that behavior analysts have taught contribute to the development of behavior that many would consider as evidence that the child has developed a theory of mind. For example, if as we suspect, being a proficient imitator leads the imitator to infer private experiences similar to one's own, then perhaps teaching generalized imitation is a component of a theory of mind. It is also likely that teaching children with autism the appropriate use of "I" and "you" pronouns aids in the development of a theory of mind, and finally, almost all attempts at teaching conventional language should develop behavior related to a theory of mind. For example, when a teacher says to a child who has a scraped knee, "That hurt," and then later when another person has a scraped knee says "That hurt," the child may come to infer that the other person is experiencing something similar to what he or she has experienced. The mechanisms which we suggest that result in children coming to make inferences about the experiences of others may be naive and completely in error. Yet, we strongly believe that behavior analysts should begin to consider how the behavior of inferring the experiences of others develops.

Summary and Conclusions

We began this paper with a review of characteristics typically ascribed to children with autism. These included such social deficits as failure to maintain eye contact, not seeking physical contact with caretakers, failure to imitate, not engaging in simple reciprocal games, failure to engage in symbolic or imaginary play, and failure to respond appropriately emotionally. Closely related to these social deficits were deficits in communication skills, including failure to demonstrate joint attention, not gesturing, communicating by mands more than tacts, failure to respond to directives and failure to develop meaningful speech. Children with autism were also more likely to exhibit stereotyped or self-stimulatory behavior, and to show rigidity in dealing with routines.

We then discussed some types of stimulus control and asked questions concerning whether limitations in stimulus control could lead to some of the characteristics of children with autism. We asked whether children with autism might differ at birth in the stimuli that control their behavior. We also asked whether the effects of certain social events, such as hugs, and other form of attention, were different for children with autism and typically developing children. We speculated that limitations in conditional discrimination learning, stimulus class learning, and recombination of stimulus-response units have major effects on a wide range of behaviors, including those which have led some to propose that children with autism have not developed an adequate theory of mind. Throughout all of our discussion of stimulus control there was a central theme that perhaps children with autism required more consistent relations between stimuli and reinforcement for stimulus control to develop. We speculated that such a requirement might explain the apparent preference of children with autism for nonsocial to social activities.

As we reviewed behavior analytic procedures used in treating children with autism, it appeared that most made a direct attempt to overcome the deficiencies listed for such children and that the procedures were primarily designed to overcome stimulus control limitations. There appeared to be an attempt throughout training to establish social praise as a reinforcer by always delivering praise on correct responses, and initially ensuring that an effective reinforcer was delivered with praise. Such a procedure seemed optimal for developing social events as conditioned reinforcers. Among the first steps in therapy programs for children with autism was the attempt to get them to look at the face of the teacher. This was done by a system of prompting and shaping with consistent reinforcement of eye contact. This procedure seemed ideal for both establishing eye contact, and establishing a person's face as a reinforcer. Soon after eye contact was established, compliance training began. This training initially began as simple successive discrimination training involving simple commands. However, it soon progressed to training involving recombination of parts of the commands. That is, training involved recombination of stimulus-response units. While the training involved a recombination of units, specific tests were not described to determine whether children could respond appropriately to commands involving new combinations. Finally, we noted that imitation and language training might attack problems related to autistic children's theory of mind. Needless to say, most of what we have presented is not new. Others have proposed behavior analytic models of autism and treatments. Since the time of Lovaas' early work, stimulus control techniques have been used in attempts to treat the behavior of autistic children. However, we hope that this paper will serve to focus research and treatment of children with autism directly on stimulus control issues.

References

Baer, D. M., Peterson, R. F., & Sherman, J. A. (1967). The development of imitation by reinforcing behavioral similarity to a model. *Journal of the Experimental Analysis of Behavior, 10*, 405-416.

Baron-Cohen, S. (1989). Perceptual role-taking and protodeclarative pointing in autism. *British Journal of Developmental Psychology, 7*, 113-127.

Baron-Cohen, S., & Swettengham, J. (1997). Theory of mind in autism: Its relationship to executive function and central coherence. In D. J. Cohen & F. R. Volkmar (Eds.), *Handbook of Autism and Pervasive Disorders* (pp. 880-893). New York: John Wiley & Sons Inc.

Bondy, A. S., & Frost, L. A. (1994). The picture exchange communication system. *Focus on Autistic Behavior, 9,* 1-19.

Brazelton, T. B., Koslowski, B., & Main, M. (1974). The origins of reciprocity: The early mother-infant interaction. In M. Lewis & L. A. Rosenblum (Eds.), *The effect of the infant on its caregiver* (pp. 49-76). New York: Wiley.

Charlop-Christy, M. H., & Kelso, S. E. (1997). *How to treat the child with autism: A guide to treatment at the Claremont Autism Center.* Claremont, California: Marjorie H. Charlop-Christy.

Curcio, F. (1978). Sensorimotor functioning and communication in mute autistic children. *Journal of Autism and Childhood Schizophrenia, 8,* 281-292.

Eikeseth, S., & Smith, T. (1992). The development of functional and equivalence classes in high-functioning autistic children: The role of naming. *Journal of the Experimental Analysis of Behavior, 58,* 123-133.

Ferster, C. B. (1961). Positive reinforcement and behavioral deficits of autistic children. *Child Development, 32,* 437-456.

Gekoski, M. J., Rovee-Collier, C. K., & Carulli-Rabinowitz, V. (1983). A longitudinal analysis of inhibition of infant distress: The origins of social expectations? *Infant Behavior & Development, 6,* 339-351.

Heimann, M., Ullstadius, E., Dahlgren, S. O., & Gillberg, C. (1992). Imitations in autism: A preliminary research note. *Behavioral Neurology, 5,* 219-227.

Kanner, L. (1943). Autistic disturbances of affective contact. *The Nervous Child, 2,* 217-250.

Keller, F. S., & Schoenfeld, W. S. (1950). *Principles of psychology.* New York: Appleton-Century-Crofts.

Krantz, P. J., & McClannahan, L. E. (in press). Social interaction skills for children with autism: A script reading procedure for beginning readers. *Journal of Applied Behavior Analysis, 31.*

Lord, C., & Rhea, P. (1997). Language and communication in autism. In D. J. Cohen & F. R. Volkmar (Eds.), *Autism and pervasive developmental disorders* (2nd ed., pp. 195-225). New York: John Wiley & Sons, Inc.

Lovaas, O. I. (1977). *The autistic child: Language development through behavior modification.* New York: Irvington.

Lovaas, I., Koegel, R. L., & Schreibman, L. (1979). Overselectivity in autism: A review of research. *Psychological Bulletin, 86,* 1236-1254.

Lovaas, O. I., & Schreibman, L. (1971). Stimulus overselectivity of autistic children in a two-stimulus situation. *Behavior Research and Therapy, 9,* 305-310.

Lovaas, O. I., Schreibman, L., Koegel, R., & Rehm, R. (1971). Selective responding by autistic children to multiple sensory input. *Journal of Abnormal Psychology, 77,* 211-222.

MacDuff, G. S., Krantz, P. J., & McClannahan, L. E. (1993). Teaching children with autism to use photographic activity schedules: Maintenance and generalization of complex response chains. *Journal of Applied Behavior Analysis, 26,* 89-97.

Mauk, J. E., Reber, M., & Batshaw, M. L. (1997). Autism and other pervasive developmental disorders. In M. L. Batshaw (Ed.), *Children with disabilities* (4th ed., pp. 425-447). Baltimore: Paul H. Brookes Publishing.

Metz, J. R. (1965). Conditioned generalized imitation in autistic children. *Journal of Experimental Child Psychology, 2*, 389-399.

Miller, J., Chapman, R., Branston, M., & Reichle, J. (1980). Language comprehension in sensorimotor Stages V and VI. *Journal of Speech and Hearing Research, 23*, 284-311.

Mundy, P., & Sigman, M. (1989). Specifying the nature of social impairment in autism. In G. Dawson (Ed.), *Autism: New perspectives on diagnosis, nature, and treatment.* New York: Guilford.

Mundy, P., Sigman, M., Ungerer, J., & Sherman, T. (1986). Defining the social deficits of autism: The contribution of nonverbal communication measures. *Journal of Child Psychology and Psychiatry, 27*, 657-669.

Osterling, J., & Dawson, G. (1994). Early recognition of children with autism: A study of first birthday videotapes. *Journal of Autism and Developmental Disorders, 24* (3), 247-257.

Papousek, H. (1992). Experimental studies of appetitional behavior in human newborns and infants. *Advances in Infancy Research, 7*, 19-53.

Rogers, S. J., & Pennington, B. F. (1991). A theoretical approach to the deficits in infantile autism. *Development and Psychopathology, 3*, 137-162.

Sidman, M. (1971). Reading and auditory-visual equivalences. *Journal of Speech and Hearing Research, 14*, 5-13.

Siegel, G. M., & Spradlin, J. D. (1978). Programming for language and communication therapy. In R. L. Schiefelbusch (Ed.), *Language intervention strategies* (pp. 357-398). Baltimore: University Park Press.

Skinner, B. F. (1957). *Verbal Behavior*, New York: Appleton, Century, Crofts.

Stone, W. L., Lemanek, K. L., Fishel, P. T., Fernandez, M. C., & Altemeier, W. A. (1990). Play and imitation skills in the diagnosis of autism in young children. *Pediatrics, 86*, 267-272.1

Thoman, E. B., Korner, A. F., & Beason-Williams, L. (1977). Modification of responsiveness to maternal vocalization in the neonate. *Child Development, 48*, 563-569.

Volkmar, F., Carter, A., Grossman, J., & Klin, A. (1997). Social development in autism. In D. J. Cohen & F. R. Volkmar (Eds.), *Handbook of Autism and pervasive developmental disorders* (Second ed., pp. 171-194). New York: John Wiley & Sons, Inc.

Wetherby, A. M., Yonclas, D. G., & Bryan, A. A. (1989). Communication profiles of preschool children with handicaps: Implications for early identification. *Journal of Speech and Hearing Disorders, 54*, 148-158.

Author Note

We wish to acknowledge the support of NICHD Grants PO1-HD-18955 and P30-HD-02528. We also wish to thank Pat White for editing the manuscript.

Discussion of Spradlin and Brady

Looking at Autism Through the Stimulus Control Window

Steven C. Hayes
University of Nevada

Behavior analysis is one of the only approaches to psychology that maintains a dynamic tension between two very distinct poles in such a thoroughgoing way. It is a source of much of the intellectual strength of the behavior tradition.

On the one hand, there is an appreciation of complexity and wholeness. The concept of an "operant" integrates a diverse range of facts under a single term. Among other things it implies a history, a setting, a set of motivational variables, and a purpose (in the descriptive sense of that term). Further, it implies the working together of all of these things, so seamlessly that the unit of analysis itself is a fusion of all of these facets.

On the other hand, there is a drive toward simplicity. There is a great deal that is known about the various facets of a behavioral interaction, although always in dynamic interaction with the other facets. Thus, there are long research traditions on such topics as stimulus control, conditioned reinforcement, or elicited behavior. When confronted with complexity, behavior analysts seek out avenues of attack based on the simpler facets of a behavioral interaction. In the hands of good behavior analysts, this interest in simplicity is not a form of reductionism. There is never a sense that the complex whole is *merely* a simpler aspect. Rather, the interest is pragmatic. Would it be useful to deal with complexity by focusing more on subsets of particular aspects and the arrangements among them than on others?

This strategy has been enormously useful. It gives behavior analysts a wide variety of lines of attack for a given problem, but without the downsides of reductionism. Stimulus control and consequential control, for example, are acknowledged to be two sides of a coin, but it may be that it is more useful to think in one set of terms as compared to another. Thus, some problems are more usefully considered to be stimulus control problems, while others are more usefully considered to be consequential problems, but at the same time there is no tendency to reify these emphases into truly separate categories.

Appreciation for both of these two poles is especially useful for applied analysts. Application almost necessarily is a matter of some complexity. Yet the wide range of basic findings in behavior analysis emerged from a pragmatic, ground-up strategy that emphasized control over simpler interactions and their aspects.

Thus, applied behavior analysts do a little dance in which they maintain an appreciation for the whole while repeatedly shifting focus to the simple (and often drawing upon the basic laboratory literature when they do so) in order to see if an advantage is acquired.

Spradlin and Brady's chapter very nicely shows these features. They are ever concerned with complexity: the wide range of clinically significant behaviors demonstrated by autistic children. I never had a sense that they were willing to forget that complexity in order to make a set of facts fit an analysis, and indeed they pushed themselves to deal with forms of complexity that most behavior analysts might be tempted to ignore (e.g., theory of mind phenomena). Yet the lens through which they examine this complexity is shockingly simple and thoroughly grounded in basis behavioral science: the ease with which stimulus control is established. In the context of this facet, a wide variety of clinical facts seem more understandable.

To my way of thinking, appreciating the coherence that comes from a given line of attack on a complex phenomenon is a first step, but only a first step. The next step of evaluation is more pragmatic: does it buy us anything new and if so is that new approach useful? Thus, the second test after apparent coherence is conceptual and technical generativity while the final test is empirical demonstrations of utility. I think Spradlin and Brady's approach was evaluated in this chapter primarily by coherence. That is a good first step, but I was less clear about what new things might flow from the analysis. I had a sense that new things would come fairly readily if the authors forced themselves to focus on what they would do differently based on their analysis. Whether all of that will then pay off is something that will need to be researched, of course.

This step (seeing what would emerge that his technically new) is also necessary because it can reveal a common problem. It is always possible that when a given analytic approach is used to generate new techniques that the apparent simplicity will collapse. That could happen here. For example, when we consider *how* to increase stimulus control we might quickly start focusing intently how to get access to powerful reinforcers. If this kind of thing happens in succession across a range of behavioral aspects then the utility of simplicity will slip away.

Metaphorically, testing out basic analyses of complex phenomena is something like looking at a complex interlocking puzzle through a multi-colored plastic cube that surrounds it. Each facet shows the puzzle in a different light. If each view inevitably leads to another ("this green window view cannot be understood unless you also look through the red, purple and yellow windows as well…and vice versa"), then it makes little difference how we initially view the puzzle. If the differences between various views are entirely aesthetic ("ah, see how it shines when we look at it through the green window"), then it likewise makes no substantive difference. But if looking at the puzzle from some facets point toward the puzzle solution more than other facets ("you can see the locking pin that holds it together, but only if you look in the green window"), then we have a difference worth emphasizing.

I am not sure yet whether viewing autistic behavior from the point of view of stimulus control is such a pragmatically useful view, although the aesthetic effect is startling enough that this seems possible. As of this moment, however, all I can say is that I enjoyed looking though the window. What I saw there seemed surprisingly coherent.

Chapter 4

Conditional Discrimination Processes, the Assessment of Basic Learning Abilities (ABLA), and their Relevance to Language Acquisition in Children with Autism

W. Larry Williams and Cynthia Reinbold
University of Nevada, Reno

This chapter describes current behavioral research and future research needs with respect to language development in children diagnosed with autism. The chapter is organized into five major areas: (1) Initial behavioral research and interventions in children diagnosed with autism; (2) Over-selectivity: A possible solution to acquisition and generalization problems. (3) The Assessment of Basic Learning Abilities (ABLA); (4) Conditional discrimination research in persons diagnosed with autism or developmental disabilities and; (5) Implications of the ABLA for current language training for children diagnosed with autism and future research

Initial Research and Interventions in Children with Autism

Autism was first described by Kanner (1943, 1944) who defined children suffering from this condition as " (a) exhibiting a serious failure to develop relationships with other people before 30 months of age, (b) problems in development of normal language, (c) ritualistic and obsessional behaviors ("insistence on sameness"), and (d) potential for normal intelligence." (Lovaas 1987 p.3)

Early attempts at treating autism were products of the "zeitgeist" of the post war era in psychology and medicine that were dominated by a psychodynamic approach. Early attempts at treating autism from this approach did not prove effective (DeMeyer, Hingtgen and Jackson, 1981; Kanner, 1943, 1944; Rimland, 1964; Rutter, 1974; Wing, 1966;)

The behavioral literature relevant to the treatment of children with autism is large enough not to permit a detailed or even comprehensive review in a short presentation. The present paper will therefore attempt to outline several major areas from the current knowledge on behavioral teaching and intervention as they developed historically to the present state of knowledge. It is hoped that such an outline of the behavioral treatment strategies to teaching language, academic and social skills to autistic children will provide both a more detailed theoretical view than was possible for Kanner in 1943 as to the nature of autism, a realistic prognosis for its treatment, and indications for research that will be necessary eventually to fully describe and understand it.

In order to achieve this goal, this paper will outline the major behavioral clinical and research approaches that have dominated activity in the area of autism over the past four decades. While the account will not attempt to be comprehensive, it will attempt to be representative.

As described by Van Houten (1990) autism was among the first developmental disorders to be treated utilising a behavioral approach. Most of the behavioral intervention literature of the sixties can be said to be representative of the "leg work" that developed methods for addressing the teaching of more complex self care, basic communication, and pre-academic repertoires that would be the first steps to autonomous functioning for autistic and other disabled children, first in institutional settings and later in community and education settings. Indeed, it was during this period of time that applied behavioral science first demonstrated the application of operant shaping and chaining methods to teach functional skills to children with autism.

The 1960s saw the development of practical intervention strategies in which the response-consequence relationship was emphasised. This is not surprising, given the focus that post war behaviourists encouraged on the response-stimulus relationships of the operant conditioning paradigm as opposed to stimulus-response relationships of Pavlovian conditioning. "Stimulus-response" psychology was very much paired for most of the academic and scientific community, albeit erroneously with the methodological behaviorism of J. B. Watson which had squandered its early influence on psychology by the end of the first half of the century. The strictness and the simplicity of its demands for dealing only with observable behavior were easily rejected for the more attractive, even if unscientific, approach to human behavior offered by the psychodynamic schools.

Early Demonstrations of Learning in Children with Autism

Many of the "breakthroughs" in securing appropriate development, education, and habilitative treatments and services for the handicapped were either prompted by, or the direct results of, individual clinical interventions, demonstration projects, and programs developed by early behavior analysts from within the educational system and the residential institutions (E.g., Allyon & Michael, 1959; Bijou & Baer 1961; Hall, Ayala, Copeland, Cossairt, Freeman & Harris, 1971; Lovass, 1966; Hall, Lund & Jackson 1968; Martin, England, Kaprowy, Kilgour & Pilek 1968, Risley & Wolfe, 1967). Early behavioral studies of the late fifties and early sixties indicated that autism as other forms of disability and learning disorder could be affected through principles of operant learning. At first simple forms of social interaction and vocalisations from young children with autism were shown to be susceptible to reinforcement (Skinner, 1954; Azrin & Lindsley, 1956; Ferster, 1961; Hingtgen & Trost 1966).

Teaching methods were devised which incorporated the original laboratory developed operant procedures of "reinforcement" (increasing the frequency of a specific behavior by arranging for consistent consequences defined as reinforcers); "extinction" (the reduction of a specific behavior due to the consistent removal of consequences which previously maintained the behavior); "shaping" (differential reinforcement of successive approximations, or, the application of reinforcement and extinction using regularly changing criteria, to establish entirely new behaviors from only initial fragments); "fading of stimulus control" (the presentation during teaching of additional gestures, vocal instructions, emphasised correct choice stimuli, etc. to aide the student in giving the right answer, and their subsequent gradual removal); "chaining" (the teaching of complex tasks by breaking them into smaller discrete behaviors, each one leading logically and functionally within the overall task to the next behavior, and then proceeding to teach each separate behavior in either a forward or reversed sequence, while arranging for each behavior to be the cue for the next behavior in the task); "modelling and imitation" (where the actual response to be performed is provided as an antecedent stimulus for the student to copy); this phenomena, of course, is the central mechanism in "social learning theory."

Of particular importance during this development was the work of Lovaas and his students in California. It was through the work of Lovaas that many of the now well established methods for teaching language and social behavior were developed (Lovaas, 1966; Lovaas, Berberich, Perloff, & Schaeffer, 1966; Lovaas, Freitas, Nelson, & Whalen, 1967; Lovaas, Schaeffer, & Simmons, 1965). These early studies clearly established that autistic symptoms could be drastically affected by consistent behavioral intervention and teaching interventions, and as we shall see, they laid the groundwork for several of Lovaas's students further to describe further the nature of learning for the child with autism.

With his early students, Lovaas, had developed one on one, trial by trial teaching procedures for establishing attention, receptive language, and to a lesser extent, expressive language in children diagnosed with autism or psychoses. These children also typically presented extreme oppositional behaviors and often severe aggression to others or themselves. A typical behavioral description of autistic symptoms, as the following derived from Lovaas, Koegel, Simmons, and Long (1973), contained more specific features:

1) Apparent sensory deficit: appear to be deaf: look and or walk through things or; normal vision when tested.
2) Severe affect isolation: fail to reach out to be picked up when approached by people; appear distant-unreachable; indifferent to being liked; are not affectionate.
3) Self-stimulatory behaviour: behaviours providing proprioceptive feedback (rocking, twirling, hand flapping, gazing, etc.
4) Mutism : 50% non- recognisable words; sounds mostly vowels.
5) Echolalia: immediate or delayed echoing of other's speech.

6) Receptive speech deficit: minimal or no receptive language.

7) Self-Help & Social skills: minimal or absence of social and self help skills; toileting, dressing, avoiding dangers, etc.

8) Self destructive or mutilatory behaviors: some display aggression to self or others; tantrums, severe oppositional behaviors.

Lovaas et al. (1973) reported one of the first long-term follow-up studies on the effects of behavior therapy with twenty children with autism. Their study was the first long-term analysis of behavioral interventions for the treatment of autism. This study (1973) represented the effects of the consistent and long-term application of the teaching methods first reported in the 1960s (Lovaas,1966; Lovaas, Berberich, Perloff, & Schaeffer, 1966; Lovaas, Freitas, Nelson, & Whalen, 1967). Their findings were that: (1) Inappropriate behaviors such as self stimulatory and echolalia, decreased during treatment, and appropriate behaviors such as appropriate speech, appropriate play, and social non-verbal behaviors increased. (2) Spontaneous social interactions and the spontaneous use of language occurred about eight months into treatment for some of the children. (3) IQs and social quotients reflected improvement during treatment. (4) There were no exceptions to improvement, however some children improved more than others did. (5) Follow-up measures recorded 1-4 years after treatment showed that large differences between groups of children depended upon the post-treatment environment (those groups whose parents were trained to carry out behavior therapy continued to improve, while children who were institutionalised regressed). (6) A brief reinstatement of behavior therapy could temporarily re-establish some of the original therapeutic gains made by the children who were subsequently institutionalised (see Lovaas et. al 1973). The initial progress had been fruitful, but there remained many problems such as attainment of more generalised repertoires, a factor calling attention to the nature of appropriate applied programming from an operant viewpoint.

With the initial demonstrations of the applicability of the operant paradigm to the behavior of challenging populations with mental illness, mental retardation, autism, and others in the 1960s (Baer, Wolf, & Risley, 1968) the way was paved for the natural emphasis that was to follow in the 1970s on the role of the antecedent stimuli in applications of the operant paradigm. Nowhere was this more apparent than in the research of those applied behavior analysts working with children with autism, and particularly in the work of the group influenced by Lovaas.

Overselectivity: A Possible Solution to Acquisition and Generalization Problems.

Lovaas, Schreibman, Koegel & Rehm (1971) introduced the term "stimulus over-selectivity". It referred to the documented observation that children with autism appeared to respond to, or come under control of, only one or two features of a multi-stimulus display. This phenomenon became more salient when it was demonstrated that typically so called "normal" children came under the control of several stimuli in a multi-stimulus presentation as a result of a typical operant discrimination teaching procedure. Children diagnosed with mental retardation appeared to respond to at least two features of the same multi-stimulus presentation, while children with autism usually came under the exclusive control, or responded exclusively to, only one feature of a multi-stimulus presentation.

The implications of this discovery quickly became staggering when researchers realised that typical "prompting" procedures in operant teaching methods would have to be re-analysed and adjusted to guard against having the learner with autism responding to irrelevant or insufficient features of multi-stimulus presentations. Such presentations would be used in even simple one-to-one instructional situations, and of course in almost all meaningful social behavior and language development. Indeed, the behavioral research into the treatment of autism in the 1970's appears to have been largely dedicated to the nature and description of over-selectivity and development of methods to circumvent it in teaching. (Lovaas & Schreibman, 1971; Koegel & Wilhelm, 1973; Schreibman, 1975; Koegel and Rincover, 1976; Koegel and Screibman, 1977; Koegel & Rincover, 1977; Rincover & Koegel, 1977).

A general method for correcting for over-selectivity was described as "within stimulus prompt fading" (Schreibman, 1975; Wolf and Cuvo, 1978), and "criterion related prompt fading" Schilmoeller & Etzel, 1977). These studies, as well as those of Rincover and his colleagues, (Anderson & Rincover, 1982; Mullins & Rincover, 1985; Rincover & Ducharme, 1987; Rincover, Feldman & Eason 1986) have since isolated many features of the autistic child's discriminatory process. This body of knowledge has shed much light on why children with autism have difficulty learning under "normal" circumstances, as well as provided insight into how to remedy as many of the variables as possible responsible for wrong, irrelevant, or lack of learning, and subsequent generalization.

Related directly to the problems for learning due to over-selectivity of stimuli is the problem of generalization. The work of Rincover and Koegel (1975, 1977) demonstrated the effects of over-selective responding in children with autism on the nature of the generalization of their responses. These collective works showed the crucial necessity for teachers of children with autism to be able to ascertain exactly which stimuli control their students responses, in order to guard against students coming under control of irrelevant stimuli or teachers' prompts during interactions. A strong implication of this knowledge is the necessity for teachers, clinicians, and family members to become aware of the actual effects of their own behaviors on the learning of children with autism. The importance of knowing exactly what we are doing when interacting with such children gained more strength as the 1970s became the 1980s, in two new and important behavioral research developments.

The Assessment of Basic Learning Abilities (ABLA)

In 1977 the journal "Rehabilitation Psychology" published a special Monograph issue (Volume 42, number 3, 1977). This monograph introduced the concept and several studies concerning a proposed hierarchy of discriminatory abilities in humans that its authors called the Auditory Visual Combined Discrimination Test (AVC) (Kerr, Meyerson, Flora, Tharinger, Schallert, Casey & Fehr, 1977). In subsequent research this test was renamed "The Assessment of Basic Learning Abilities" (ABLA). Although the work was developed with persons with mental retardation, it had and continues to have great relevance for learners with autistic features or a diagnosis of autism.

The ABLA basically demonstrates through a 30 minute set of simple one-to-one teaching trials, whether someone can imitate, make a visual discrimination of position, a visual discrimination along some dimension between two objects, a simple conditional visual discrimination (matching to sample), a simple auditory discrimination, and a conditional auditory-visual discrimination. Since the late 1970s, several researchers have investigated a theoretical hierarchy of six levels of visual and auditory discriminations that both normal children and those with DD and Autism appear capable of making (Casey & Kerr, 1977; Fehr & Kerr, 1977; Meyerson & Kerr, 1977, Kerr, Meyerson, & Flora, 1977; Meyerson, 1977; Tharinger, Schallert, & Kerr, 1977; Martin, Yu, Quinn, & Patterson, 1983; Wacker, Steil, & Greenbaum, 1983; Yu, Martin & Williams 1989).

The ABLA hierarchy includes four levels of visual discrimination (1) imitation, (2) position, (3) physical dimension (e.g., color, size, and shape), and (4) matching to sample (the ability to pair visually similar objects). Two subsequent levels involve audio discrimination, (5) simple auditory discrimination, and (6) auditory-visual conditional discrimination. In a table-top situation, the test materials include a large yellow open can, a similar sized red open square box, two pieces of randomly shaped foam, a small yellow cylinder, and a small red cube. A person's ability to demonstrate or acquire the above discriminations is determined in less than one hour, following a set protocol (see Kerr, Meyerson & Flora, 1977; Yu, Martin, & Williams, 1989).

The early work in this area by Kerr et al. demonstrated that (1) there does appear to be a hierarchy of discriminatory difficulty at least within persons with mental retardation, and that hierarchy is described by the ABLA test. That is, persons who fail a given level on the test typically fail all levels above that level. (2) Levels that appear to be frequently problematic for learners with developmental disabilities are the simple auditory level, and the conditional auditory/visual level. That is, persons with developmental disabilities often can make conditional visual discriminations, but have difficulty in making auditory-visual conditional discriminations. (3) Normal educational development and language require ABLA discriminations.

Initial research that followed Kerr et al. (1977) consisted of replications and verifications of the general findings. Yu, Martin & Williams (1989) provided a review of this work. Extensions had been made with children diagnosed with autism (Rossito, 1984) indicating that the ABLA test is relevant for this population also. Further implications of the test as demonstrated by Williams, Rossito, Dal'Acqua, Schurachio, Figueirdo, Esteves, Fuimaraes, Macedo, & Alves (1983) were that both autistic and mentally retarded children who were followed for over two years and tested regularly on the Portage guide to early education (Blume, Shearer, Froham, & Hillard, 1976) as a measure of development, showed consistent inability to pass developmental test items which required ABLA skills at levels beyond those that they showed on independent ABLA tests. These outcomes gain more significance if one considers the misleading cues for a diagnosis of mental retardation versus infantile autism in the pre-school child. Meyers (1989) has argued that infantile autism is more likely to be diagnosed than mental retardation in children with the same performance due to prognosis variables. Meyers argues that most children with infantile autism are also mentally retarded, while many severely retarded children show autistic tendencies. Although some work had been conducted in teaching children to make discriminations at levels they initially could not make, (Meyerson & Kerr, 1977) many successful reports indicated the effective role of "within stimulus prompting" methods (Witt & Wacker, 1981) as well as emphasising response-reinforcer relationships and using response prevention methods (Glen, Whaley, Ward & Buck, 1980; Yu & Martin, 1986).

More recent research has demonstrated that there may be interim levels of visual discrimination, especially conditional visual discriminations, as well as interim conditional auditory discriminations that once acquired, have resulted in some subjects acquiring auditory skills they were previously shown to not have (Barker-Collo, 1995; Harapiak, Martin, & Yu, (1998); Lin, Martin, & Collo, 1995; Walker, Graham, DeWiele, & Martin, 1989; Walker & Martin, 1989; Walker, Lin, & Martin, 1994; Ward, 1995; Cummings & Williams, 1997), as well as the predictive utility of the ABLA (McDonald & Martin, 1993; Stubbings & Martin, 1995).

Walker, Lin, and Martin (1994) examined whether it might be valuable to add an additional diagnostic task to the ABLA hierarchy. The task that may be worth adding is the assessment of the ability to make an auditory match-to-sample discrimination. Whereas all levels of the ABLA appear to be important, the ability to make auditory discriminations may be the most important of all. One contributing factor may be that the ABLA test, as currently structured, is missing a critical skill between level 4, visual match-to-sample, and level 5, auditory discrimination. The missing level may be that of auditory match-to-sample.

The results clearly support the positioning of the auditory identity, matching task in the ABLA hierarchy between level 4 and level 5. All subjects who passed level 5 also passed the auditory matching test. All of those who failed the visual discrimination and lower on the ABLA test also failed auditory matching. If auditory matching is an intermediary step between ABLA levels 4 and 5, then we would expect that some who pass up to and including level 4 would pass auditory identity matching, while others who pass up to but not including level 4 would fail auditory identity matching.

Perhaps the presence of auditory matching skills in a subject's repertoire might be the missing ingredient that makes it easier for a subject to learn auditory discriminations. If subjects who pass the test of auditory identity matching but fail level 5 are able to learn a two-choice auditory discrimination more quickly than subjects who fail both the test of auditory identity matching and level 5, then it may be worthwhile to teach auditory identity matching skills as a prerequisite to the learning of two-choice auditory discriminations.

Barker-Collo (1995) compared performance on the ABLA test to that on three live-to-live speech sound matching tasks, and three live-to-live simple sound matching. Comparison of speech and simple sound task performance would allow exploration of the suggestion that speech sounds are more difficult to learn than simple sounds. Her results indicated: a) ability to match live-to-live auditory cues is more difficult than ABLA level 6; and b) individuals passing live-to-live simple sound matching tasks will also pass live-to-live speech sound matching tasks. Live-to-live auditory matching is more difficult than ABLA level 6. This implies that live-to-live auditory matching may be potential addition to the ABLA test. One difference between ABLA level 6 and live-to-live auditory matching is the complexity of auditory cues. The added complexity of the sounds presented in live-to-live simple and speech sound matching tasks may increase task difficulty. Increased task difficulty may also be due to the absence of visual cues.

In live-to-live auditory matching, the position of the matching sound is randomly alternated over trials; however, no visual cues are made available to aid in determining the correct response, as simple sounds are made behind visual shields and lip movements are hidden from view.

Individuals unable to pass live-to-live simple sound matching tasks were also unable to pass speech sound matching tasks. This indicates that speech and simple sound matching tasks may exist at the same level of difficulty if all other elements remain equal. These results appear to contradict previous claims that speech sounds are more difficult for individuals with developmental disabilities to learn than simple sounds. Barker–Collo suggested that further research should be conducted to determine whether live-to-live auditory matching adds to our ability to predict classroom learning and ability to perform prevocational analogue tasks. Future research may also focus on development of training procedures which allow individuals currently passing ABLA level 6 who fail live-to-live auditory matching tasks to learn these failed tasks.

Lin, Martin, and Collo (1995) proposed that an auditory matching task might be a prerequisite to learning more complex auditory discriminations. Differences emerged in the subjects they studied between the difficulty of matching live-to-taped speech sounds versus live-live speech sounds. Auditory matching appears to be involved in everyday situations such as recognizing individuals by the sound of their voice, repeating words spoken by others, recognizing successive instances of the telephone ringing, and whispering when others are whispering versus shouting when others are shouting. Second, the ability to perform an auditory matching task may be important to facilitate learning of more complex auditory discriminations. These results extend the predictive validity of the auditory matching test beyond the results reported by Walker et al. (1994). Firstly, participants in Group 1 who failed the auditory matching test (and ABLA levels 5 and 6) also failed to match common sounds and live-to-taped speech sounds. The participants in Group 2 who passed the auditory matching test (but failed ABLA levels 5 and 6) were also able to match common sounds and live-to-taped speech sounds. Secondly, matching common sounds and live-to-taped speech sounds appears to be easier than both auditory discriminations (levels 5 and 6) and live-to-live speech sound matching. More research with this method is needed. Considering the potential benefits of mastering all levels on the ABLA test including the auditory matching test, Lin, Martin & Collo suggested future research might focus on four areas: 1) studies might examine ways to program generalization of auditory matching ability across a variety of auditory matching tasks; 2) research is needed to asses the value of testing auditory matching as a prerequisite to teaching levels 5 and 6 on the ABLA test to participants who have failed these level; 3) the difficulty of live-to-live speech sound matching relative to level 6 on the ABLA test might be further explored; 4) research might explore the differences in antecedents and consequences between live-to-live and live-to-taped auditory matching in order to isolate the variable(s) that determine differences in difficulty between these tasks.

Harapiak, Martin, and Yu (1998) expanded the ABLA to include four additional auditory discriminations and examined the hierarchical ordering of the new discriminations. Two lines of evidence suggest that it may be worthwhile to examine the relationship between the ABLA auditory tasks and other types of auditory discriminations. First, the ability to pass the ABLA auditory tasks may be prerequisite to learning more complex language discriminations. Second, research indicates that failed ABLA auditory discriminations are extremely difficult to teach using standard prompting and reinforcement procedures, often requiring hundreds of training trials.

Harapiak et al. suggested further types of auditory discriminations: One type involves hearing a sound, and then responding to an apparatus to produce the same sounds. Another type of auditory discrimination involves hearing three sounds, two of which are identical (or very similar), and indicating which of the two sounds are identical.

They employed the following testing procedures: 1) a two-choice task to produce a matching sound; 2) a two-choice task to produce a non-matching sound; 3) auditory - auditory identity matching; 4) auditory-auditory nonidentity matching. The results, in conjunction with those of Walker et al. (1994), Lin et al. (1995), and Ward (1995) provided strong evidence that the bell-tambourine (a two choice task to produce a matching sound) task falls between ABLA levels 4 and 6, and that two of the other three auditory matching tasks are hierarchically ordered beyond ABLA level 6.

The practical implication of these findings is that it allows further differentiation of clients previously grouped as ABLA level 6. The authors suggested that future research might replicate the study with a larger number of participants, as well as attempt to determine the extent to which ABLA levels 5 and 6 and the four auditory matching tasks in this study are related to measures of communication abilities.

Vause, Martin, and Yu (in Press) reported on a different use of the ABLA for persons with DD. This study demonstrated that there was a higher frequency of aberrant responses during training sessions with training tasks above or below a participant's assessment level on the ABLA test. The present study extended previous research in that the ABLA test provided a reliable method for measuring task difficulty and learning ability for persons with developmental disabilities. Several studies indicate that there is considerable potential for use of multiple-component training packages for teaching failed two-choice visual and auditory discriminations. The present study suggests that a portion of training time would be valuably spent if devoted to tasks that have a difficulty level that matches the highest ABLA test level of that client. These results are consistent with those reported earlier by Sayrs, Wilder, & Williams, (1995) and Empy, Wilder, Higbee, Williams, Martin, & Bennett (1995) in which the ABLA was administered as part of a pre-treatment functional analysis of aggressive behavior in two adult males with DD. The results of these analyses showed that aggression functioning as escape from demand was significantly reduced when instructions were made using visual (signs and symbols) rather than auditory modalities (spoken). The participants had previously been shown to be non-responsive to auditory stimuli, having failed on the ABLA at levels 5 & 6.

In summary, current research supports and furthers the original proposition by Kerr et al. (1977) for a hierarchy of visual and auditory discrimination abilities. To date, no study has shown subjects who, having failed at one level of discrimination skill, demonstrate higher level skills. Importantly, a common observation is that subjects with developmental disabilities or autism-spectrum features often have difficulty learning conditional visual discriminations (level 4 of the ABLA), and then do not demonstrate simple auditory or conditional auditory-visual discriminations (levels 5 & 6 of the ABLA). These kinds of discriminations are crucial to normal language development and subsequent complex reasoning skills. Indeed, as we have seen, a major observation about persons with mental retardation or autism centers on their difficulty or inability effectively to respond to either complex visual stimulus relations, or relations between stimuli that are from different sensory modalities (auditory and visual). Whereas the bulk of the ABLA research has verified the hierarchical relationship of visual discriminations, (levels 1, 2, & 3) conditional visual discriminations (level 4), auditory discriminations (level 5), and auditory-visual discriminations (level 6), the recent studies (e.g., Harapiak, Martin & Yu, 1998) have supported the possible existence of interim levels of visual, auditory, and auditory-visual discrimination. As many of the discriminations involved in the typical ABLA levels represent differing combinations of the features that define different and well identified types of conditional discriminations, we will now turn to an analysis of research that has examined conditional discrimination processes in persons with developmental disabilities or autism.

Conditional Discrimination Research in Persons with Autism or Developmental Disabilities

A basic discrimination is said to have occurred when a learner comes to respond in the presence of a given environmental event or stimulus (discriminative stimulus) and not when it is absent. The discrimination develops as a result of a reinforcing consequence (reinforcer) consistently occurring only following occurrences of the response in the presence of the discriminative stimulus and not in its absence. A conditional discrimination is one which represents a logical "if-then" rule with respect to the relationship between stimuli wherein "a response to a given stimulus is followed by a reinforcer if and only if another stimulus is present" (Green, Mackay, McIlvane, Saunders, & Soraci, Jr. (1990) (p. 250). For example, learning to point to a green object in the presence of the vocal statement "green" is a conditional discrimination in which a pointing response has come under the conditional control of the stimulus "green" (as opposed to "red" or other sounds). Conditional discriminations may occur within and across any sensory modality. They have been studied for many years with animals and more recently with humans, as they represent the basic building blocks of concepts and or rules (Dixon & Dixon, 1978; Sidman & Tailby, 1982). For a review of the early, basic laboratory, conditional discrimination research the reader is referred to Carter and Werner (1978). Spradlin and Brady (this volume) provide a description of the role of complex conditional discriminations and their resulting stimulus control in children diagnosed with autism.

In investigating the nature of conditional discrimination processes, many variables have been examined. Typically, the variables have been examined using a procedure known as "matching-to-sample," in which a subject is required to respond to one of at least two comparison (choice) stimuli depending on the prior presentation of a specific stimulus (sample). Thus, a given stimulus is chosen conditional upon a previous stimulus, and the eventual discrimination established is a conditional discrimination. Within such an arrangement, procedural variables such as how physically similar (e.g., color, size, shape, weight, etc.) or otherwise related (relationship or function) the sample and the choice stimuli are; whether the sample remains present during the choosing of the comparison stimulus; when the sample is removed before the comparisons are presented, the delay between the termination of the sample and the presentation of the comparison stimuli; whether the comparison stimuli are presented simultaneously or successively to each other; and the sensory modality of any of the stimuli are some of the variables that have been investigated. While space does not permit an extensive review of this literature, our purpose is to relate several, representative findings of the current literature.

Green et al. (1990) describe and define conditional discrimination, conditional stimulus relations and stimulus equivalence, generalized stimulus relations, accounts of emergent behavior (mediation by other responses), and relational learning and memory (mediated remembering and levels of processing). Despite research conducted over the past 40 years, there has yet to emerge a systematic set of procedures for teaching people with DD to respond to relations among stimuli. They argue that whereas improvements have been made; 1) there is not a large amount of collective experience in teaching relational discriminations to individuals who lack substantial language skills; 2) there have been substantial and impressive successes in individual cases that, taken at face value, suggest that careful training can overcome problems associated with low functional level; and 3) it is not unreasonable to consider the great success that has been achieved in teaching animals, subjects who are unarguably nonverbal.

Saunders & Spradlin (1989) have shown that the acquisition of matching-to-sample performances can be facilitated by procedures that explicitly require a) successive discriminations among the sample stimuli; b) simultaneous discrimination among the comparison stimuli; and c) likely to influence acquisition is the requirement that discriminative functions of the comparison stimuli change from trial to trial. Further work by these researchers (Saunders & Spradlin 1990, 1993) has demonstrated the effectiveness of standard simple discrimination training with reversals, and the blocking of trials in which the same sample comparison relations are presented for many (blocks) of trials and then gradually reduced over trials until they are presented randomly.

Saunders, Williams, & Spradlin (1995) found that new arbitrary matching-to-sample problems require learning specific sample-comparison relations, which in turn requires the successive discrimination of the sample stimuli (responding differentially to stimuli that never appear together). In contrast, when identity is a basis for responding, specific sample-comparison relations need not be learned (Stromer and Stromer, 1989) and stimuli need only be discriminated simultaneously.

McIlvane, Dube, Kledaras, Iennaco, & Stoddard (1990) described efforts to devise new procedures that might teach relational discriminations more effectively. Their programming methodology made use of what has been learned about stimulus shaping, the development of learning set, and the formation of stimulus classes based on relations with consequences.

Dube, Green, & Serna (1993) provided data indicating that many failures to demonstrate same/different judgments in low-functioning individuals were likely due to methodological limitations of extant test procedures. Serna, Dube, and McIlvane (1997) reported a series of studies which has led to a principle technology for assessing same/different judgments in low-functioning individuals with mental retardation.

They examined previous attempts over the past decade to teach same/different judgments to individuals with mental retardation and age equivalent scores below 5 years. Stimulus-control shaping procedures, including fading and delayed prompting, minimal intervention procedures, and the proceeding procedures supplemented with the 3-stage programmed method constituted these attempts. Dube, Moniz, and Gomes (1995) asked whether a computer-delivered fading procedure would be as effective as a human teacher's verbal and nonverbal prompts for teaching new visual discriminations to individuals with DD. Both types of instruction were effective with some subjects, and neither was effective with all subjects.

Their results indicated: a) on trials where prompts were given, the teacher prompts were effective with more subjects than was the computer-fading procedure; and b) when computer fading was effective, transfer to task stimuli was nearly perfect. In contrast, effective teacher prompts typically led to poor stimulus control transfer.

Some research has specifically addressed differences in visual and auditory-visual discrimination. Green (1990) reported on 5 young adult females with mild MR who were given match-to-sample training and testing to develop four classes of equivalent stimuli (Sidman & Tailby, 1982). For 4 of the 5 subjects, the classes that included auditory stimuli developed more rapidly than those that did not. All subjects eventually demonstrated the emergence of two visual and two auditory-visual equivalence classes of three stimuli each following training on conditional relations in each class. For 3 of 5 subjects, the equivalence relations emerged more quickly in the auditory-visual case. These results were consistent with those reported by Sidman et al. (1986). Together these studies suggest reliable differences in the formation of auditory-visual and all visual classes, at least when subjects are learners with mental retardation. An important question for future research is whether the differences in formation of auditory-visual and visual-visual classes will be observed only in persons with mental retardation.

Kelly, Green, and Sidman (in press) provide evidence that successful auditory-visual matching does not guarantee proficiency in visual-visual identity matching. An initial screening test yielded a surprising pattern: the participant did considerably better at auditory-visual matching than visual-visual identity matching. The subject's success in auditory-visual matching demonstrated that he was capable of discriminating the visual stimuli. However, he performed poorly on a visual-visual identity matching task. His problem, therefore, had to lie either in learning relations between visual samples and visual comparisons, or in some aspect of the teaching and testing procedures, or in both of these. Subsequent success in teaching the participant to do identity matching demonstrated that his earlier deficient performances had not arisen from a visual-visual relational deficit. A critical aspect of testing procedures turned out to be the number of comparison stimuli that were presented on each trial. When the child worked with an equal number of stimuli that were used in the testing phase he was able to maintain a high level of visual-visual identity matching, and to generalize this skill to new stimuli.

This study demonstrated that a participant's ability to match auditory samples to visual comparisons does not guarantee an ability to do identity matching with those same visual stimuli. Although visual discrimination is a prerequisite for auditory-visual matching, visual-visual matching involves many factors other than stimulus discriminations, including procedural features that generate or require behavior that the reinforcement contingencies do not specify explicitly, such as selection of positive or rejection of negative comparisons, and effective scanning of the display. It will not do to assume that cross modal matching implies adequate identity matching under the particular procedures that one is using.

Table one is here presented in an effort to clarify for the reader the possible combinations of procedures involved in identity versus arbitrary conditional relations, as well as whether sample and/or comparison stimuli are presented simultaneously or successively.

The table attempts to present six possible arrangements for establishing conditional discriminations for each of three modality situations: visual, auditory,

Table 1.Procedural Variations in Establishing Conditional Discriminations.

(* Indicates correct choice)

	Identity		Arbitrary	
	SAMPLE	COMPARISON	SAMPLE	COMPARISON
1. Identity	green red	green* red*	4. green red	red* green*
2. Simultaneous Sample-comp	green red	.green*, green, red .green, red, red*	5. green red	green, green, red* green*, red, red
3. Successive Sample-comparson	green red	green*red green,red*	6. Green red	green, red* green*red
1. Identity	buzz ring	buzz* ring*	4. buzz ring	ring* buzz*
2. Simultaneous Sample-comp	buzz ring	buzz*, buzz, ring buzz, buzz, ring*	5. buzz ring	buzz, buzz, ring* buzz*, buzz, ring
3. Successive Sample-comp	buzz ring	buzz*, ring buzz, ring*	6. buzz ring	buzz, ring* buzz*, ring
1. Identity	green red	buzz* ring*	4. green red	buzz* ring*
2. Simultaneous Sample-comp	green red	buzz*,green, ring buzz, red, ring*	5. green red	buzz*, green, ring buzz, red, ring*
3. Successive Sample-comp	green red	buzz*, ring buzz, ring*	6. green red	buzz*, ring buzz, ring*

Note:
1. Interim procedures involving timing of presentations are not shown.(e.g., simultineity of comparson stimuli as opposed to sample and comparison stimuli, and auditory samples as opposed to only visual for auditory-visual discriminations) .
2. Note that Auditory levels 2 & 5 rarely occur in everyday life except in complex musical types of situation, similarly for levels 3 & 6 as both would be presented simultaneously. Many examples could be given for these auditory levels if we consider the comparisons being presented successively (as noted above).
3. The variables of "arbitrary" and "cross modality" (Auditory-visual) render such discriminations at least equally difficult- all other factors held constant.

and auditory-visual. The table assumes the simplest of situations in which a sample stimulus is presented, and then comparison stimuli are presented for a choice to be made. At the first level, a learner is required to select the stimulus presented when presented again (identity), and only that stimulus is presented as a comparison. At the second level, a stimulus is presented, and then is presented again with two choice stimuli. In identity matching, the sample stimulus is considered correct, whereas in arbitrary matching Levels 4, 5, & 6) a specific new stimulus is correct. At a third level, only the comparison choice stimuli are presented. These can be presented immediately, and either at the same time, or in any combination of delay, increasing the difficulty of the task accordingly.

Several features of the possible procedures become salient upon examination. In the auditory section, it is hard to provide typical daily discrimination examples where we are required to choose between two or more comparison stimuli that are presented simultaneously. Indeed, such situations are typically aversive, and we arrange for the successive presentation of such stimuli in order better to attend to them (e.g., two people speaking at once). It is also easy to see from the table that auditory-visual discriminations are by definition arbitrary discriminations. This feature of cross modality discrimination, that is, its arbitrariness, needs analysis as to its additional difficulty as compared for example to the simultaneous or successive presentation of comparison or sample and comparison stimuli. Notice, for example, that the auditory-visual identity and arbitrary presentations are identical at this simplest of analyses. If new stimuli were added the complexity is increased. In an attempt to organize the relevant research on the ABLA, and that work that is relevant from basic conditional discrimination research along the relations described in table one, tables two, three, and four describe conditional discriminations as represented in the ABLA test. These discriminations are for visual, auditory and auditory-visual stimuli that are identity or arbitrary in nature, and involve simultaneous or successive presentations of stimuli that are of simple or multiple dimensions.

Several representative studies on conditional discrimination and/or stimulus equivalence, conducted with persons with autism or developmental disabilities, as well as articles describing subsets of discrimination skills for the original ABLA hierarchy, are located on the tables. Obviously not all possible relevant independent variables can be represented in such tables. For example, the number and location of sample and choice stimuli, reinforcement delivery procedures, component stimulus features and their location in stimuli used, or general session procedures are included. There was also no attempt to include gustatory, olfactory or tactile discriminations. However, a comparison of the mode (visual, auditory, auditory-visual combined) and whether the procedure was identity or arbitrary matching compared to the simultaneity or successive nature of the stimulus presentations, allows for a visual representation of the relevant current literature.

An immediate feature of the tables is that there is logical support for the ABLA hierarchy, as well as the work that has produced interim skills, with relation to other

Table 2. Features of Conditional Visual Discriminations

	Simultaneous		Successive			
	Single Dimension	Multiple Dimension	Single Dimension Short Delay	Single Dimension Long Delay	Multiple Dimension Short Delay	Multiple Dimension Long Delay
Modality: Visual						
Identity	Imitation –2 Position –2 Form –3 Match –4 *Examples:* McIlvane et al. (1990)	Imitation-1 Form-3 Match-4 ABLA Levels 1-4 *Examples:* Kerr and Meyerson (1977)	*Examples:* Stromer et al. (1993) Saunders et al. (1994) Dube et al. (1992)		*Examples:* Stromer et al. (1993)	
Arbitrary	*Examples:* Ward (1995) McIlvane et al. (1990) Saunders & Spradlin (1989) Green (1990) Calcagno et al. (1994) Dube et al. (1995)	*visual equivalence* PECS 2D-3D	*Examples:* Saunders & Spradlin (1989) (1990) (1993)	*visual equivalence*	*Examples:* McIlvane et al. (1990)	*visual equivalence*

Table 3. Features of Conditional Auditory Discriminations

| | Simultaneous | | | | Successive | |
	Single Dimension	Multiple Dimension	Single Dimension Short Delay	Single Dimension Long Delay	Multiple Dimension Short Delay	Multiple Dimension Long Delay
Modality: Auditory						
Identity	Examples: Walker et al. (1994)		*Vocal Imitation (sounds & single words)* Examples: Harapiak et. al (1998)	*Vocal Imitation (phrases)*		
Arbitrary	Examples: Ward (1995)		*Audio equivalence* Examples: Lin et al. (1995) Dube et al. (1993) Vause et al. (Submitted)		*ABLA audio-5* *Simple Instruction*	

Table 4. Features of Conditional Auditory-Visual Discriminations

	Simultaneous		Successive			
	Single Dimension	Multiple Dimension	Single Dimension Short Delay	Single Dimension Long Delay	Multiple Dimension Short Delay	Multiple Dimension Long Delay
Modality: Auditory-Visual Identity			*ABLA Level 5* (black & white)		Examples: Lin et al. (1995) Harapiak et al. (1998) Barker-Collo (1995) Kelly et al. (In press) Walker et al. (1994)	
Arbitrary	*Simple receptive object Labeling* Examples: Ward (1995) Eikeseth & Smith (1992) Harapiak et al. (1998)	Summers et al. (1993) Examples: Green (1990)	*Delayed receptive object labeling* ABLA Level 6 (black & white)	*Expressive & receptive action phrases*	*ABLA Level –6* Examples: Partington et al. (1994) Walker et al. (1994) Eikeseth & Smith (1992) *Auditory-Visual equivalence* Sidman & Tailby (1982)	*Language* Examples: Barker-Collo (1995) Harapiak et al. (1998)

research on conditional discrimination in persons with autism or developmental disability. In terms of difficulty, or hierarchy, it is clear that one proceeds from top (visual) to bottom (auditory-visual) and then from left (simultaneous) to right (successive). Whether auditory discrimination appearing to follow visual discrimination is due to the methodological (successive) nature of auditory discriminations, or to some other feature, has yet to be established. However, evidence is mounting for this ordering of human operant discrimination skills.

Implications of the ABLA for Current Language Training for Children with Autism and Future Research

Intensive discrete trial training methods have increased in recent years since the original documented interventions with this population in the 1960s (Beukelman & Mirenda, 1993; Charlop, Schreibman & Thibodeau, 1985; Charlop & Walsh, 1986: Harris & Handleman, 1994; Koegel & Koegel, 1995; MacDuff, Krantz, & McClannahan, 1993; Maurice, Green & Luce, 1996; Quill, 1995; Schreibman, 1988; Siegel, 1996). Central to all methods is an intensive effort to establish and expand communication abilities that are a major skill deficit observed in persons with autism and other developmental disabilities. Most approaches include teaching procedures that have been developed to overcome the difficulty that many learners have in making discriminations in situations in which complex multiple stimuli are presented, such as are involved in language acquisition (Partington, Sundberg, Newhouse, & Spengler, 1994; Sigafoos & Reichle, 1992). These methods are the result of previous research that clarified the ways in which many learners respond in an over selective manner to stimulus presentations that involve multiple cues or dimensions (Lovaas & Schreibman, 1971; Lovaas, Schreibman, Koegel, & Rehm, 1971; Reynolds, Newsom, & Lovaas, 1974; Schreibman, 1975; Wilhelm & Lovaas, 1976; Lovaas, Koegel, & Schreibman, 1979; Rincover, Feldman, & Eason, 1986; Rincover, & Ducharme, 1987; Summers, Rincover, & Feldman, 1993). While these approaches have enhanced teaching many more children to acquire many concepts and communication abilities, the establishment of vocal communication remains one of the major difficulties in this population (Maurice et al 1996; Quill, 1995).

Current language training in autism typically initially promotes vocal imitation, progressing to receptive and then expressive skills (Beukelman & Mirenda, 1993; Maurice et al., 1996; Siegel 1996). One popular approach to establishing communication in children with autism has been to establish a Picture Exchange Communication System (PECS) (Bondy, 1996; Bondy & Frost, 1994, 1995). This method has the child learn to choose a picture of an object and exchange it for the object. Thus a non-vocal communication system is established which may then lead to eventual vocal communication. Regardless of the picture system used, the final performance can be seen to involve arbitrary matching to sample, where the picture (a two dimensional object) is associated with the actual three-dimensional object. Dixon (1981) has shown that persons with DD or autism may not respond to pictures of objects as representations of those objects, but rather as separate three-dimensional objects. In terms of what we have discussed previously with respect to ABLA levels, it may be that matching a picture of an object with the object represents a conditional visual discrimination that is more complex than the task of matching actual objects to other actual objects, especially if the objects are identical. Ward (1995) demonstrated that some subjects who were not capable of passing ABLA level 5 (simple auditory) acquired that skill after training on more complex visual conditional discriminations.

Vocal imitation can be viewed as involving conditional identity auditory matching. That is, although other (expressive) skills are involved, one cannot emit a sound and adjust it to match a given sound, without being able to match the sounds auditorially. Lin, Martin & Collo (1995) and Harapiak et al. (1998) have reported data that indicate that discrimination of identical sounds may precede the same task using voices that are taped, or when human live voices are not identical but arbitrary as in ABLA levels 5 & 6.

Cummings & Williams (1997) reported acquisition data for five children with autism who received in home discrete trial training of varying amounts per week. All the children received training almost daily on visual matching to sample, vocal imitation, and the picture exchange communication system (PECS). They observed that the PECS system was typically mastered within a varying number of trials after, but never before, a child had passed a learning criterion of 3 consecutive ten trial blocks at 80% correct on a real object matching to sample task. In turn, they observed that vocal imitation (a task they argued can be seen to involve at least identity auditory matching) "emerged" only after each child passed the same learning criterion for matching pictures to real objects on the PECS training (a task they argued represents a complex visual conditional discrimination). Although these results do not conflict with any of the known literature, they present further perplexing questions concerning the sufficient and necessary conditions under which subjects may acquire certain conditional discriminations. They prompt further investigation into the role of teaching procedure and method versus pre-requisite skills for more complex discriminations, and await further replication.

Related to the above discussion is the role of "manding" (Skinner 1957) in the promotion of further verbal behavior acquisition. It may be, for example, that in a communication system such as PECS engaging in behavior that results in consequences that are of immediate relevance for a child (manding involves verbal behavior that specifies environmental changes that satisfy a current state of deprivation or that remove a current relative aversive state), may promote further and different functioning forms of verbal behavior. Thus, it may be the manding function of the PECS training that promotes vocal imitation, as opposed to the analysis provided by Cummings & Williams (1997). For a comprehensive discussion of the relevance of a behavior analytic "verbal behavior" approach to research in language acquisition in children with autism see Sundberg and Partington's chapter on language training.

Another feature of the ABLA test involves the actual materials and protocol used. Whereas the original intent of the ABLA authors was to provide ample opportunity for a subject to demonstrate his or her discrimination ability at any given level, by providing materials that allowed a discrimination to be made in any of several dimensions, this feature may work against some learners given the over-selectivity literature. As an example, consider the materials used for level 4 (visual matching to sample). In a table-top situation, a large yellow open can, a similar sized red open square box, a small yellow cylinder, and a small red cube are used in a two-choice matching to sample procedure. However, whereas one can readily admit a similarity between a large yellow open topped, metal can and a small wooden yellow cylinder, or a red, square, open topped box, and a small red wooden cube, one could just as easily see that these objects differ along any number of dimensions. Just how different do stimuli have to be to render a discrimination task as arbitrary rather than identity? Could subjects be "hooking" on an irrelevant but differing feature of these objects and not discriminating their similarities? Given the analysis we have provided on the apparent hierarchical nature of a variety of conditional discriminations, both within and across modalities, control of such variables as identity versus arbitrary would seem important (c.f. Stromer, McIlvane, Dube, & MacKay, 1993). In an attempt to answer such questions, we are currently undertaking an examination of the ABLA by using materials that are black & white (to eliminate color blindness) and that differ only along one dimension at a time.

Finally, research is needed on verifying the possible relationships between discriminations made across different sensory modalities. While some work has been reported (e.g., O'Leary & Bush, 1996), questions as to the relationship of auditory discriminations to tactile and olfactory levels, and these in turn to visual discriminations, remain.

References

Anderson, N.A., & Rincover, A. (1982). The generality of overselectivity in developmentally disabled children. *Journal of Experimental Child Psychology*, *34*, 217-230.

Ayllon, T. & Michael, J. (1959). The psychiatric nurse a behavioral engineer. *Journal of the Experimental Analysis of Behavior*, *2*, 323-334.

Azrin, N., & Lindsey, O.R. (1956). The reinforcement of cooperation between children, Journal *of Abnormal and Social Psychology*, *52*, 100-102.

Baer, D.M., Wolf, M., & Risley, T. (1968) Some current dimensions of applied behavior analysis. *Journal of Applied Behavior Analysis*, *1*, 91-97.

Barker-Collo, S. (1995). Live-to-live auditory matching: An extension of the Assessment of Basic Learning Abilities Test? *Developmental Disabilities Bulletin*, *23*, 72-81.

Beukelman, D. R. & Mirenda, P. (1993). *Augmentative and Alternative Communication: Management of severe communication disorders in children and adults*. Baltimore, MD: Paul H Brookes.

Bijou, S. W. & Baer, D. M. (1961). *Child Development: A systematic and empirical theory*, Vol.1. New York: Appleton-Century-Crofts.

Bluma, S., Shearer, M., Frohman, A., & Hilliard, J. (1976). *The Portage Guide to Early Education*. (Rev. ed.) Portage, Wisconsin: Co-operative Educational service Agency, No.12.

Bondy, A. (1996). What parents can expect from public school programs. In Catherine Maurice, Gina Green, & Stephen Luce, (Eds.). *Behavioral Intervention for Young Children with Autism: A Manual for Parents and Professionals*. Austin, Texas: Pro-ed.

Bondy, A. & Frost, G. (1994). The Picture-Exchange Communication System. *Focus on Autistic Behavior, 9*, 1-19.

Bondy, A. & Frost, G. (1995). Educational approaches in preschool: Behavioral techniques in public school setting. In E. Schopler & G. Mesibov (Eds.), *Learning and cognition in autism* (pp. 311-333). New York: Plenum.

Carter, D. E., & Werner, T. (1978). Complex learning and information processing by pigeons: a critical analysis. *Journal of the Experimental Analysis of Behavior, 29*, 565-601.

Casey, M. and Kerr, N. (1977). Auditory-visual discrimination and language production. *Rehabilitation Psychology, 24*,137-155.

Charlop, M. H., Schreibman, L., & Thibodeau, M. G. (1985). Increasing spontaneous verbal responding in autistic children using a time delay procedure. *Journal of Applied Behavior Analysis, 18*, 155-166.

Charlop, M. H. & Walsh, M. E. (1986). Increasing autistic children's spontaneous verbalizations of affection: An assessment of time delay and peer modelling procedures. *Journal of Applied Behavior Analysis, 19*, 307-314.

Cummings, A. & Williams, W. L. (1997). Emergence of functional vocal verbal communication in autistic children: An analysis of a picture exchange communication system. Poster presentation at the 23rd annual meeting of the Association for Behavior Analysis, Chicago.

DeMeyer, M.K., Hingtgen, J.N., & Jackson, R.K. (1981). Infantile Autism reviewed: A decade of research. *Schizophrenia Bulletin, 7*, 388-451.

Dixon, L. (1981). A functional analysis of photo-object matching skills of severely retarded adolescents. *Journal of Applied Behavior Analysis, 14*, 465-478.

Dixon, M. H., & Dixon, L. S. (1978). The nature of standard control in children's matching-to-sample. *Journal of the Experimental Analysis of Behavior, 30*, 205-212.

Dube, W. V., Green, G., & Serna, W. (1993). Auditory successive conditional discrimination and auditory stimulus equivalence classes. *Journal of the Experimental Analysis of Behavior, 59*, 103-114.

Dube, W.V., Moniz, D. H., and Gomes, J.F. (1995). Use of computer and teacher delivered prompts in discrimination training with individuals who have mental retardation. *American Journal of Mental Retardation, 100*, 253-261.

Empy, C, Wilder, D., Higbee, T., Williams W. L., Martin, C. & Bennett, M. (May 1996). Functional analysis and intervention in a case of severe aggression. Paper presented in the symposium W.L. Williams (chair) Analysis and Intervention in community services for the developmentally disabled. 22nd annual meeting of the Association for Behavior Analysis, San Francisco.

Fehr, M., & Kerr, N. (1977). Auditory discrimination and language. *Rehabilitation Psychology, 24*, 156-168.

Ferster, C. B. (1961). Positive reinforcement and behavioral deficits of autistic children. *Child Development, 32*, 437-456.

Ferster, C.B. & De Meyer, M.K. (1961). The development of performances in autistic children in an automatically controlled environment. *Journal of Chronic Diseases, 13*, 312-345.

Glenn, S. S., Whaley, D. L., Ward, R. & Buck, R. W. (1980). Obtaining color discriminations in developmentally disabled children by disrupting response stereotyping. *Behavior Research of Severe Developmental Disabilities, 1*, 175-189.

Green, G. (1990). Differences in development of visual and auditory-visual equivalence relations. *American Journal on Mental Retardation, 95*, 3, 250-270.

Green, G., Mackay, H. A., McIlvane, W. J., Saunders, R. R., & Soraci, S.A. (1990). Perspectives on relational learning in mental retardation. *American Journal on Mental Retardation, 95*, 249-259.

Hall, R.V., Ayala, H., Copeland, R., Cossairt, A., Freeman, J., & Harris, J. (1971). Responsive teaching: An approach for teaching teachers in applied behavior analysis techniques. In A. Ramp and B.L. Hopkins (Eds.), *A new direction for Behavior Analysis*, Kansas, University of Kansas.

Hall, R.V., Lund, D., & Jackson, D. (1968). Effects of teacher attention on study behavior. *Journal of Applied Behavior Analysis, 1*, 1-12.

Harapiak, S. M., Martin, G.L., and Yu, D. (submitted for publication). Hierarchical ordering of auditory discriminations and the assessment of basic learning abilities test.

Harris, S.L., & Handleman, J.S. (1994). *Preschool education programs for children with autism*. Austin, Texas: PRO-ED.

Hingtgen, J.N. & Trost, F.C, (1966). Shaping co-operative responses in early childhood schizophrenics: Reinforcement of mutual physical contact and vocal responses. In R. Ulrich, T. Stachnik, & J. Mabry (Eds.) *Control of Human Behavior*, Vol. 1., Glenview. Ill: Scott, Forseman Co.

Kanner, L. (1943). Autistic disturbances of affective contact. *Nervous Child, 2*, 217-250.

Kanner, L. (1944). Early Infantile Autism. *Journal of Paediatrics, 25*, 211-217.

Kelly, S., Green, G., & Sidman, M. (In press). Visual identity and audio-visual matching: A procedural note. *Journal of Applied Behavior Analysis*.

Kerr, N., Meyerson, L., & Flora, J. (1977). The measurement of motor, visual and auditory discrimination skills. *Rehabilitation Psychology, 24*, 95-112.

Kerr, N., Meyerson, L, Flora, Tharinger, Schallert, Casey, & Fehr (1977). The measurement of motor, visual, and auditory discrimination skills. *Rehabilitation Psychology, 24,* 91-94.

Koegel, R.L., & Koegel, L.K. (1995). *Teaching children with autism.* Baltimore: Paul H. Brookes.

Koegel, R.L., & Wilhelm, H. (1973). Selective responding to the components of multiple visual cues by autistic children. *Journal of Experimental Child Psychology, 15,* 442-453.

Koegel, R. L., & Rincover, A. (1976). Some detrimental effects of using extra stimuli to guide learning in normal and autistic children. *Journal of abnormal Child Psychology, 4,* 59-71.

Koegel, R.L., & Rincover, A. (1977). Research on the difference between generalization and maintenance in extra-therapy responding. *Journal of Applied Behavior Analysis, 10,* 1- 12.

Koegel, R, L., & Schreibman, L. (1977). Teaching autistic children to respond to simultaneous multiple cues. *Journal of Experimental Child Psychology, 24,* 299-311.

Lin, Y.H., Martin, G. L., & Collo, S. (1995). Prediction of auditory matching performance of developmentally handicapped individuals. *Developmental Disabilities Bulletin, 23,* 1-15.

Lovaas, O.I. (1966). A program for the establishment of speech in psychotic children. In J.K. Wing, (Ed.), *Early Childhood Autism (pp. 115-144),* Elmsford, N.Y., Pergamon Press.

Lovaas, O. I. (1987). Behavioral treatment and normal educational and intellectual functioning in young autistic children. *Journal of Counseling and Clinical Psychology, 55,* 3-9.

Lovaas, O.I., Schaeffer, B., & Simmons, J.Q. (1965). Building social behaviors in autistic children by use of electric shock. *Journal of Experimental studies in Personality, 1,* 99-109.

Lovaas, O.I., Berberich, J.P., Perloff, B.F., & Schaeffer, B. (1966). Acquisition of imitative speech in Schizophrenic children. *Science, 151,* 705-707.

Lovaas, O.I., Freitas, S., Nelson, K., & Whalen, C. (1967). Building social and preschool behaviors in schizophrenic and autistic children through non-verbal imitation training. *Behavior Research and Therapy, 5,* 171-181.

Lovaas, O.I., Koegel, R., & Schreibman, L. (1979). Stimulus overselectivity in Autism: A review of research. *Psychological Bulletin, 86,* 1236-1254.

Lovaas, O.I., & Schreibman, L. (1971). Stimulus overselectivity of autistic children in a two stimulus situation. *Behavior Research and Therapy, 9,* 305-310.

Lovaas, O.I., Schreibman, L., Koegel, R, & Rehm, R. (1971). Selective responding by autistic children to multiple sensory input. *Journal of Abnormal Psychology, 77,* 211-222.

Lovaas, O.I., Koegel, R., Simmons, J Q., & Long, J.S. (1973). Some generalization and follow up measures on autistic children in Behavior Therapy. *Journal of Applied Behavior Analysis, 6,* 131-165.

MacDuff, G. S., Krantz, R.L., & McClannahan, L.E. (1993). Teaching children with autism to use photographic activity schedules: Maintenance and generalization of complex response chains. *Journal of Applied Behavior Analysis, 26,* 89-9.

McDonald, L. & Martin, G. L. (1993). Facilitating discrimination learning for persons with developmental disabilities. *International Journal of Rehabilitation Research, 16,* 160-164.

Martin, G. L., England, G., Kaprowy, E., Kilgour, K., & Pilek, V. (1968). Operant conditioning of kindergarten-class behavior in autistic children. *Behavior Research and Therapy, 6,* 281-294.

Martin, G., Yu, D., Quinn, G., & Patterson, S. (1983). Measurement and training of AVC discrimination skills: Independent confirmation and extension. *Rehabilitation Psychology, 28,* 231-237.

Maurice, C., Green, G., & Luce, S. C. (1996). *Behavioral intervention for young children with autism: A manual for parents and professionals.* Austin, Tx: Pro-ed.

McIlvane, W.J., Dube, W. V., Kledaras, J. B., Iennaco, F.M., & Stoddard, L. T. (1990). Teaching relational discrimination to individuals with mental retardation: Some problems and possible solutions. *American Journal on Mental Retardation, 95,* 283-296.

Meyers, B. A. (1989). Misleading cues in the diagnosis of mental retardation and infantile autism in the pre-school child. *Mental Retardation, 27,* 85-90.

Meyerson, L. (1977). AVC behavior and attempts to modify it. *Rehabilitation Psychology, 24,* 119-122.

Meyerson, L. & Kerr, N. (1977). Teaching auditory discriminations to severely retarded children. *Rehabilitation Psychology, 24,* 123-128.

Mullins, M. & Rincover, A. (1985). Comparing Autistic and normal children along the dimensions of reinforcement maximization, stimulus sampling, and responsiveness to extinction. *Journal of Experimental Child Psychology, 40,* 350-374.

O'Leary, C. A. & Bush, K. M. (1996). Stimulus equivalence in the tactile modality. *The Psychological Record, 46,* 509-517.

Partington, J. W., Sundberg, M. L., Newhouse, L., and Spengler, S.M. (1994). Overcoming an autistic child's failure to acquire a tact repertoire. *Journal of Applied Behavior Analysis, 27,* 733-734.

Quill K.A. (1995). *Teaching children with autism: Strategies to enhance communication and socialization.* New York: Delmar

Reynolds, B., Newsom, C. & Lovaas, O.I. (1974). Auditory overselectivity in autistic children. *Journal of Abnormal Child Psychology, 2,* 253-263.

Rimland, B. (1964). *Infantile Autism.* New York: Appleton-Century Crofts.

Rincover, A., & Ducharme, J. M. (1987). Variables influencing stimulus overselectivity and "tunnel vision" in developmentally delayed children. *American Journal of Mental Deficiency, 91,* 422- 430.

Rincover, A., Feldman, M., and Eason, R. (1986). "Tunnel vision": Variables influencing stimulus control in autistic children. *Analysis and Intervention in Developmental Disabilities, 6,* 283-304.

Rincover, A. & Koegel, R. L. (1975). Setting generality and stimulus control in autistic children. *Journal of Applied Behavior Analysis, 8,* 235-246.

Rincover, A., & Koegel, R. L. (1977). Research on the education of autistic children: recent advances and future directions. In B.B. Lahey & A. Kazdin (Eds.), *Advances in Clinical Child Psychology.* Vol.1. New York: Plenum Press.

Risley, T. R., & Wolf, M. M. (1967). Establishing functional speech in echolalic children. *Behavior Research and Therapy, 5,* 73-78.

Rossito, A. L. (1984). A comparative study of the Portage Guide to Early Education and the AVC scale: Implications for programming pre-school activities for exceptional children. Unpublished Masters thesis, Federal University of Sao Carlos, Sao Paulo, Brazil.

Rutter, M. (1974). The development of infantile autism. *Psychological Medicine, 4,* 147-163.

Saunders, K. J., & Spradlin, J. E. (1989). Conditional discrimination in mentally retarded adults: The effect of training the component simple discriminations. *Journal of the Experimental Analysis of Behavior, 52,* 1-12.

Saunders, K. J., & Spradlin, J. E. (1990). Conditional discrimination in mentally retarded adults: The development of generalized skills. *Journal of the Experimental Analysis of Behavior, 54,* 239-250.

Saunders, K. J., & Spradlin, J. E. (1993). Conditional discrimination in mentally retarded subjects: Programming acquisition and learning set. *Journal of the Experimental Analysis of Behavior, 60,* 571-585.

Saunders, K.J., Williams, D.C., & Spradlin, J. E. (1995). Conditional discrimination by adults with mental retardation: Establishing relations between physically identical stimuli. *American Journal on Mental Retardation, 99,* 558-563.

Sayrs, D., Wilder, D., & Williams, W. L. (May 1995). Analysis and intervention involving antecedent condition manipulations in a pre-vocational day program for persons with developmental disabilities. Paper presentation in the symposium W.L. Williams (Chair). Changing Challenging Behavior by Altering Antecedent Environmental Conditions at the 21st annual convention of the Association for Behavior Analysis, Washington.

Schilmoeller, K.J., & Etzel, B. C. (1977). An experimental analysis of criterion related and non-criterion-related cues in errorless stimulus control procedures. In B.C. Etzel, J.M. LeBlanc, & D.M. Baer (Eds.), *New Developments in behavior research: Theory, Method and Application.* (pp.317-347). Hillsdale, N.J: Erlbaum.

Schreibman, L. (1975). Effects of within-stimulus and Extra-stimulus prompting on discrimination learning in autistic children. *Journal of Applied Behavior Analysis, 8,* 91-113.

Schreibman, L. (1988). *Autism.* Newbury Park, CA: Sage

Serna, R. W., Dube, W. V., & McIlvane, W. J. (1997). Assessing same/different judgments in individuals with severe intellectual disabilities: A status report. *Research in Developmental Disabilities, 18*, 343-368

Sidman, M., Willson-Morris, M., and Kirk, B. (1986). Matching-to-sample procedures and the development of equivalence relations: The role of naming. *Analysis and Intervention in Developmental Disabilities, 6*, 1-19.

Sidman, M., & Tailby, W. (1982). Conditional discrimination vs. matching to sample: an expansion of the testing paradigm. *Journal of the Experimental Analysis of Behavior, 37*, 5-22.

Siegel, B. (1996). *The World of the Autistic Child: Understanding and Treating Autistic Spectrum Disorders.* New York: Oxford University Press

Sigafoos, J. & Reichle, J. (1992). Comparing explicit to generalized requesting in an augmentative communication mode. *Journal of Developmental and Physical Disabilities, 4*, 167-188

Skinner, B.F., (1954) A new method for the experimental analysis of the behavior of psychotic patients. *Journal of Nervous and Mental Disorders, 120, 403-406.*

Skinner, B. F. (1957). *Verbal Behavior.* Acton, Mass: Copley.

Stromer, R., McIlvane, W. J., Dube, W., V., & MacKay, H. A. (1993). Assessing control by elements of complex stimuli in delayed matching to sample. *Journal of the Experimental Analysis of Behavior, 59*, 83-102.

Stromer, R. & Stromer, J. B. (1989). Children's identity matching and oddity: Assessing control by specific and general sample-comparison relations. *Journal of the Experimental Analysis of Behavior, 51*, 47-64.

Stubbings, V. and Martin, G.L. (1995). The ABLA test for predicting performance of developmentally disabled persons on prevocational training tasks. *International Journal of Practical Approaches to Disability, 19*, 12-17.

Summers, J., Rincover, A., & Feldman, M. (1993). Comparison of extra-stimulus and within-stimulus prompting to teach prepositional discriminations to preschool children with developmental disabilities. *Journal of Behavioral Education, 3*, 287-298.

Tharinger D., Schallert, D. & Kerr, N. (1977). Use of AVC tasks to predict classroom learning in mentally retarded children. *Rehabilitation Psychology, 24*, 113-118.

Van Houten, R. (1990). Autism. In J. M. Matson (Ed.), *Handbook of Behavior Modification with the Mentally Retarded.* New York: Plenum Press.

Vause, T., Martin, G.L., and Yu, D. (Submitted for publication). Aberrant behavior of persons with developmental disabilities as a function of the characteristics of training tasks.

Wacker, D., Steil, D., & Greenbaum, F. (1983). Assessment of discrimination skills of multiply handicapped preschoolers and prediction of classroom task performance. *Journal of the Association of the severely handicapped, 8*, 65-78.

Walker, J., Graham, M., DeWiele, L., & Martin, G. (1989, October). Auditory identity matching: A possible addition to the AVC discrimination test. Poster presented at the 5th annual conference of AAMR region VIII, Winnipeg, Manitoba.

Walker, J., Lin, Y.H., & Martin, G. L. (1994). Auditory matching skills and the ABLA test: where do they fit? *Developmental Disabilities Bulletin, 22,* 1-15.

Walker J., & Martin, G. L. (May 1989). Teaching auditory discriminations to a severely handicapped individual. Poster presented at the 15th annual meeting of the Association for Behavior Analysis, Milwaukee, Wisconsin.

Ward, R. (1995). Bridging the gap between visual and auditory discrimination learning in children with severe developmental disabilities. Unpublished Doctoral Dissertation: University of Toronto.

Wilhelm, H., & Lovaas, O.I. (1976). Stimulus over selectivity: A common feature in autism and mental retardation. *American Journal of Mental Deficiency, 81,* 26-31.

Williams, W. L. & Cummings, A. R. (Submitted for publication). Arbitrary visual matching to sample may lead auditory identity matching (Vocal Imitation).

Williams, W. L., Rossito, A.L., Dal'Acqua, M.J., Schurachio, M.A., Figueiredo, A.J., Esteves, M. G., Guimaraes, C.S.O., Macedo, S. E., & Alves J. M. (1983). Programmed instruction for developmentally delayed pre-school children: The experimental pre-school at PMEE-APAE in Sao Carlos. Paper presented at the annual meeting of the Psychological Society of Rebeirao Preto.

Wing, J.K., (1966). *Early Childhood Autism:* Elmsford, N.Y. Pergamon Press.

Witt, J., & Wacker, D. (1981). Teaching children to respond to auditory directives: An evaluation of two procedures. *Behavior Research of Severe Developmental Disabilities, 2,* 175-189.

Wolfe, V. F., & Cuvo, A.J. (1978) Effects of within-stimulus and extra-stimulus prompting on letter discrimination by mentally retarded persons. *American Journal of Mental Deficiency, 83,* 297-303.

Yu, D., & Martin, G. L. (1986). Comparison of two procedures to teach visual discriminations to severely mentally handicapped persons. *Journal of Practical Approaches to Developmental Handicaps, 10,* 7-12.

Yu, D., Martin, G. L., & Williams, W. L. (1989). Expanded Assessment for discrimination learning with mentally retarded persons: A practical strategy for research and training. *American Journal of Mental Retardation, 94,* 161-169.

Discussion of Williams and Reinbold

Establishing Communicative Repertoires in Disabled Persons

Ruth Anne Rehfeldt
University of Nevada, Reno

Williams and Reinbold describe a training procedure that is intended ultimately to establish a vocal imitation repertoire in individuals with few or no initial echoic skills. This procedure is based on the notion that the mastery of a theoretical hierarchy of six levels of visual and auditory discriminations is critical for effective communicative abilities. The protocol known as the Assessment of Basic Learning Abilities (ABLA) contends that an individual's failure to learn the discriminations at any level will result in an observed failure to demonstrate the discriminations required by higher levels of the hierarchy. Williams and Reinbold focus on the final three levels of this hierarchy, in which visual-visual conditional discrimination learning precedes auditory-visual conditional discrimination learning, and which may represent at a simple auditory conditional discrimination level the development of imitative vocal responses.

According to Cummings & Williams (1997), five developmentally disabled children were trained conditionally to relate identical two-dimensional objects. At the same time, they received training to relate symbolically three-dimensional and two-dimensional objects as a component of the Picture Exchange Communication System. Vocal imitation was also trained concurrently during these sessions. The performance of all five children indicated that vocal imitation was established only after some level of the picture exchange task (visual-visual complex conditional discrimination learning) was mastered, which likewise improved dramatically after the children had performed successfully on the identity matching-to-sample (visual-visual simple conditional discrimination learning) tasks. In addition, the spontaneous emission of words was displayed by some of the children following their demonstration of correct imitation. Cummings & Williams (1997) conclude speculatively that visual-visual conditional discrimination skills (trained at level 4 of the hierarchy) may be prerequisites for vocal imitation, or the demonstration of auditor-auditory identity relations.

Williams and Reinbold's account of this promising research program is noteworthy in that it gives rise to a number of important theoretical and practical questions. Clearly their discussion holds important implications for understanding the role of conditional discrimination learning in language acquisition, why failures or difficulties to establish conditional discriminative control may be common among developmentally disabled persons, and how such failures might be remedied.

Necessary Repertoires

When highly specific training histories lead to the emergence of novel and desirable topographies, there is much cause for excitement concerning the nature of that history. In this case, the required history for vocal imitation appears to be extended training in complex visual-visual conditional discrimination learning. Interestingly, the apparent requirement that visual-visual conditional discrimination skills be intact before an individual can master auditory-visual conditional discrimination skills stands in contrast to a body of results which suggests that auditory-visual conditional discriminations may actually be established with greater ease than visual-visual conditional discriminations. Several studies to date have shown that auditory-visual matching-to-sample training procedures, in which subjects learn to match dictated words to pictures or printed words, may be more effective than visual-visual matching-to-sample training procedures in several ways: First, auditory-visual procedures may require less training time to establish baseline conditional relations than visual-visual procedures; second, the emergence of equivalence classes following auditory-visual training procedures may be observed over fewer test trials than the emergence of equivalence classes following visual-visual training procedures; and third, some subjects may perform with higher accuracy on equivalence tests following auditory-visual training procedures than following visual-visual training procedures (e.g., Green, 1990; Lipkens, Hayes & Hayes, 1993; Sidman, 1971). One possible explanation for these results is that individuals with limited repertoires are likely to relate visual objects on the basis of formal, as opposed to functional, properties of the objects, a strategy which is less likely if the stimuli are of different modalities. If a repertoire of making visual-visual conditional discriminations is required before an individual can demonstrate exemplary performance on auditory-visual conditional discrimination tasks, this is difficult to reconcile with the literature indicating that auditory-visual conditional discrimination training procedures may be more effective. Is it possible that individuals who demonstrate greater success rates with auditory-visual procedures have already mastered the six levels of the ABLA hierarchy of skills?

A related issue concerns the continued attempts of behavior analysts to clarify the role of verbal names for stimuli which enter into symbolic relations with one another. It has been suggested that when objects are established as discriminative for an individual's naming of that object, the name may then occasion appropriate listener action with respect to the object and other objects (Horne & Lowe, 1996). It is further suggested that this repertoire is sufficient for the subsequent emergence of conditional relations between visual stimuli, as a consequence of the stimuli sharing membership in the same name relation (Horne & Lowe, 1996; Stromer & MacKay, 1996). Again, the rationale underlying the ABLA and the authors' data suggest that these repertoires may develop in a reverse order. It is doubtful that the subjects in the present report were able to name objects prior to training, since they did not even demonstrate echoic behavior. Do the present data refute the notion that verbal names play a critical role in conditional discrimination learning? Further work in this area may be theoretically important for purposes of contributing to resolutions of this timely issue.

Future Investigations

There are two other potentially valuable areas of investigation that might elucidate how the ABLA protocol engenders novel performances. First, the picture-exchange task requires individuals, upon the therapist's request, to hand the therapist a picture of a desired object in exchange for the actual object. This training involves the strengthening of the mand repertoire. It may be profitable to explore how mand training might give rise to echoic performance. Mands are reinforced by character-istic consequences that are specified in the mands themselves (Skinner, 1957, p. 35-36), but reinforcement for echoic behavior may take other forms. Specifically, echoic behavior may be reinforced when it brings the speaker into continued perceptual contact with the object and allows him or her to respond to it in other ways (Skinner, 1957, p. 57). How these two verbal operant classes are related in the present report is unclear, but through continued research in this area, more may be learned about the conditions under which a particular verbal operant class is ac-quired.

Second, the implications of the reported data for the sensory impaired may merit appraisal. Individuals with blindness, for example, are incapable of mastering visual-visual conditional discrimination tasks, yet clearly the responding of such persons does come under auditory discriminative control. Just how such persons master the final level of the hierarchy is currently unexplained. It seems reasonable to suspect that control by stimuli of other modalities may enable sensory impaired persons to advance through the six levels of the hierarchy. Emergent conditional relations have been observed with stimuli of modalities other than visual and auditory. Hayes, Tilley, and Hayes (1986) demonstrated the establishment of equiva-lence classes using gustatory stimuli, for example; Bush (1993) noted the establish-ment of conditional relations between auditory and tactile stimuli, reporting also that auditory-visual conditional discriminations were extended to tactile stimuli that resembled visual stimuli in form and size (see also O'Leary & Bush, 1996). Whether the learning of conditional relations between stimuli of other, less-fre-quently investigated modalities is sufficient for the establishment of communica-tion skills is an important question with respect to designing and implementing training programs for the sensory impaired.

To conclude, Williams and Reinbold have ventured into a research arena that is wide open for the resolution of a number of practical and theoretical issues. More research will be useful in assessing the utility of ABLA in teaching individuals communicative skills, as well as further clarifying some of the theoretical issues that have been raised. Replications of the reported data, as well as controlled laboratory studies, would be promising avenues to pursue in our continued attempts to understand the interplay between conditional discrimination learning and language processes.

References

Bush, K. M. (1993). Stimulus equivalence and cross-modal transfer. *The Psychological Record, 43*, 567-584.

Cummings, A. & Williams, W.L. (1997, May). Emergence of functional vocal verbal communication in autistic children: An analysis of a picture exchange communication system .children. Poster presentation at the 23rd annual meeting of the Association for Behavior Analysis, Chicago.

Green, G. (1990). Differences in the development of visual and auditory-visual equivalence relations. *American Journal on Mental Retardation, 95*, 260-270.

Hayes, L. J., Tilley, K. L., & Hayes, S. C. (1986). Extending equivalence class membership to gustatory stimuli. *Psychological Record, 38*, 473-482.

Horne, P. J., & Lowe, C. F. (1996). On the origins of naming and other symbolic behavior. *Journal of the Experimental Analysis of Behavior, 65*, 185-242.

Lipkens, R., Hayes, S. C., & Hayes, L. J. (1993). Longitudinal study of the development of derived relations in an infant. *Journal of Experimental Child Psychology, 56*, 201-239.

O'Leary, C. A. & Bush, K. M. (1996). Stimulus equivalence in the tactile modality. *The Psychological Record, 46*, 509-517.

Sidman, M. (1971). Reading and auditory-visual equivalences. *Journal of Speech and Hearing Research, 14*, 5-13.

Skinner, B. F. (1957). *Verbal Behavior*. New York: Appleton-Century-Crofts.

Stromer, R., & MacKay, H. (1996). Naming and the formation of stimulus classes. In T.R. Zentall & P.M. Smeets (Eds.), *Stimulus class formation in humans and animals* (pp. 21-252). Amsterdam, The Netherlands: Elsevier.

Chapter 5

Identifying and Assessing Reinforcers Using Choice Paradigms

Cathleen C. Piazza, Wayne W. Fisher, Lynn G. Bowman, and Audrey Blakeley-Smith
Kennedy Krieger Institute
and Johns Hopkins University School of Medicine

The identification of reinforcing stimuli for persons with developmental disabilities such as autism is an important aspect of both behavior acquisition and behavior reduction programs. That is, the effectiveness of programs designed to facilitate the acquisition of skills may be highly dependent upon the identification and use of potent reinforcers. In addition, the success of positive reinforcement programs designed to decrease maladaptive behavior (e.g., differential reinforcement of other behavior schedule [DRO]) may be effective only when the reinforcers used are potent.

Identification of potent reinforcers for persons with autism remains a significant challenge for a number of reasons. First, impairments in communication represent one of the defining characteristics of autism. Thus, the ability of persons with autism to express wants and needs may be limited. Therefore, verbal report (e.g., Cautela & Kastenbaum, 1967; Homme, Csanyi, Gonzales, & Rechs, 1969), a primary strategy used to identify reinforcers with other populations, often may not be effective for persons with autism. Second, individuals with autism often have a restricted range of interests and activities. Thus, direct observation of behavior may not be informative regarding preferences if few behaviors are spontaneously emitted during the observation period. A third related difficulty is that frequently occurring behavior may be aberrant (e.g., stereotypy, self-injurious behavior, aggression) and may not be appropriate to use as a reinforcer. Finally, some persons with autism may have limited exposure to pleasurable events in the environment for a variety of reasons (e.g., placement of an individual in a restrictive environment), and thus the client may not respond to some activities due to a lack of familiarity with those events.

Most studies on reinforcer identification have focused on either: (a) identifying potential reinforcers (i.e., stimulus preference assessments) without testing whether or to what extent the stimuli could be used to increase a response (e.g., Cautela & Kastenbaum, 1967; Homme et al., 1969); or (b) assessing the reinforcing effects of stimuli (i.e., reinforcer assessments) without a procedure for predicting which specific stimuli would function as reinforcers (e.g., Dattilo, 1986; Wacker, Berg, Wiggins,

Muldoon, & Cavanaugh, 1985). A major advance in the identification of reinforcers for persons with disabilities occurred when Pace, Ivancic, Edwards, Iwata, and Page (1985) integrated a simple, straightforward procedure for identifying preferred stimuli based on direct observation of approach responses combined with a method for quickly assessing whether preferred stimuli actually functioned as reinforcers.

The single-item presentation method described by Pace et al. (1985) consists of two steps. First, an assessment of stimulus preference is conducted. During the stimulus preference assessment, a standard set of stimuli representing various sensory consequences is presented to the client. The dependent variable is client approach responses (e.g., looking at or manipulating the item). The client is presented with each item individually, and his or her approach responses result in brief access to the item. The results of the stimulus preference assessment can be used to construct a hierarchy of preferred stimuli. The second step of the procedure is the reinforcer assessment in which the reinforcing effects of stimuli are assessed. During the reinforcer assessment, rates of behavior (typically simple target responses such as head turning) are compared under free operant (baseline) and reinforcement conditions. In the reinforcement condition, access to the preferred stimuli identified during the preference assessment is provided contingent on the target response. The advantage of using the procedure described by Pace et al. is that the stimulus preference assessment can be used to evaluate a large number of stimuli (e.g., 16) in a time-efficient manner in order to predict which items will function as reinforcers. By contrast, the reinforcer assessment procedure is less time efficient because only a few stimuli (e.g., one or two) can be evaluated simultaneously. Thus, without the stimulus preference assessment, multiple stimuli may need to be evaluated using the more time consuming reinforcer assessment method in order to identify reinforcing effects.

One limitation of the single-item presentation method is that its accuracy may be compromised in cases where clients consistently approach all or many stimuli. In these cases, clients may approach items simply because items are presented; thus, not all approach behaviors may represent preference responses. Therefore, Fisher et al. (1992) extended the work of Pace et al. (1985) by comparing the single-item presentation method with a choice method of stimulus presentation. In the Fisher et al. study, 4 clients were exposed to an assessment in which stimulus items were presented in pairs, and an assessment in which stimulus items were presented individually. Client approach responses (i.e., pointing at, looking at, orienting toward a specific stimulus) were used as a measure of preference during both procedures. The results of the two preference assessments were then compared using a concurrent operants arrangement in which clients had access to two different stimuli. One stimulus was identified as highly preferred by the single-item presentation method, but not by the choice assessment. The other stimulus was identified as highly preferred by both the choice and single-item presentation methods. The results showed that the choice assessment resulted in greater differentiation among stimuli, and better predicted which items would function as reinforcers when compared to the single-item presentation method.

In the Pace et al. (1985) and Fisher et al. (1992) studies, the presented stimuli were chosen from a standard list of items representing various sensory categories (e.g., vestibular, kinesthetic). One question proposed by Fisher and colleagues was whether more potent reinforcers could be identified using items generated by caregiver report. Previous investigators (e.g., Green, Reid, Canipe, & Gardner, 1991; Green et al., 1988) reported that caregiver report inconsistently resulted in the accurate identification of reinforcers. Therefore, Fisher, Piazza, Bowman, and Amari (1996) developed a structured interview called the Reinforcer Assessment for Individuals with Severe Disabilities (RAISD) in order to improve the accuracy of caregiver report. The RAISD was designed to obtain verbal information on stimuli from a variety of domains, including: (a) visual, (b) auditory, (c) olfactory, (d) tactile, (e) gustatory, (f) sensori-motor, (g) social attention, and (h) toys. For example, to obtain information regarding auditory stimuli, a caregiver would be asked,

"Some children really enjoy different sounds such as listening to music, car sounds, whistles, beep, sirens, clapping, people singing, etc. What are the things you think _____ most likes to listen to?"

The authors then evaluated the extent to which information from the RAISD could be integrated with a choice assessment (Fisher et al., 1992) to improve reinforcer identification.

In the first phase of the investigation, client-preferred items were nominated by caregivers using the RAISD. Caregivers then rank ordered the predicted preferences of the client from most to least preferred. Caregivers also predicted their client's preferences of the standard list of items used by Pace et al. (1985). Fisher et al. (1996) found that correlations between caregiver predictions of client preference and the results of the choice assessment were not statistically significant when a standard set of items was used ($r = .19$). However, the correlation between caregiver predictions and the results of the choice assessment were statistically significant when the items identified through the RAISD were used ($r = .32$; $p < .005$). However, the correlation between the results of the RAISD and the choice assessment were low suggesting that use of the RAISD, in absence of a choice assessment, may not result in accurate reinforcer identification.

In the second part of this investigation, Fisher et al. (1996) evaluated whether reinforcer identification could be improved by using items from the RAISD in combination with the choice assessment. Two choice assessments were conducted with all clients, one with stimuli based on caregiver report using the RAISD and one with the 16 standard stimuli from the Pace et al. (1985) investigation. Highly preferred items (items approached on over 80% of trials) were identified based on the results of each choice assessment (i.e., highly preferred caregiver items and highly preferred standard items). The authors then conducted a reinforcer assessment comparing highly preferred caregiver items with highly preferred standard items using a concurrent operants method. In the concurrent operants method, two identical target responses were available (e.g., sitting in chair A versus chair B). One of these responses (e.g., sitting in chair A) resulted in access to the caregiver item and the other response (e.g., sitting in chair B) resulted in access to the standard item.

For all 5 clients, higher levels of responding were associated with the caregiver-selected stimulus. The results of the investigation suggested that (a) caregivers are not very accurate at predicting client preferences for items from a standard list; (b) caregivers are slightly more accurate at predicting client preference for items identified through the RAISD; and (c) a choice assessment identified more potent reinforcers when the items assessed were generated through caregiver report using the RAISD, than when items were used from a standard list.

Previous studies on reinforcer identification have shown that highly preferred items (generally identified as those items approached on 80% or more of trials) function as reinforcers. However, the extent to which the degree of preference varies systematically with reinforcer efficacy has only recently been evaluated. Piazza, Fisher, Hagopian, Bowman, and Toole (1996) assessed whether the results of a choice assessment predicted relative reinforcer effectiveness. Stimuli were categorized as high, medium, and low preference based on the results of choice assessments conducted with 4 clients. The reinforcing effects of these categories of stimuli were then compared using a concurrent operants method. High-preference stimuli were defined as those ranked first, second, and third in the choice assessments; medium-preference stimuli were the three items closest to the median (usually those ranked 7th, 8th, and 9th); and low-preference stimuli were usually those ranked 13th, 14th, and 15th. In 2 of the 4 clients, high-preference stimuli always functioned as reinforcers; medium-preference stimuli functioned as reinforcers, but only when compared to low-preference stimuli; and low-preference stimuli never functioned as reinforcers. For the remaining 2 clients, high-preference stimuli consistently functioned as reinforcers; however, medium- and low-preference stimuli failed to function as reinforcers. These data suggest that a choice assessment was accurate in predicting the relative reinforcing value of stimuli.

In the stimulus choice assessment described by Fisher et al. (1992), 16 items were compared. Each stimulus was presented with every other stimulus for a total of 120 trials. Treadwell, Fisher, and Amari (1994) evaluated whether caregiver rankings of stimuli generated by the RAISD could be used to decrease the length of the choice assessment without significantly sacrificing accuracy. First, 16-item choice assessments were completed with 20 clients. The authors then evaluated the level of agreement between the full choice assessment and briefer versions of the assessment containing 12, 8, and 4 items. Two different methods of selecting the items for the briefer choice assessments were compared. With one method, items were selected based on caregiver rankings from the RAISD. With the other method, items were repeatedly selected at random using Monte Carlo statistical analyses (i.e., to determine the levels of agreement expected by chance). When items were selected using the results of the RAISD, agreement levels between the brief and full choice assessments exceeded chance expectation. For example, the agreement level between the 8-item choice assessment and the 16-item choice assessment was 80% (i.e., 80% of the items identified as high preference by the full assessment also were identified as high preference by the 8-item assessment). Thus, the length of the choice assessment was decreased by 78%, but the agreement with the full choice assessment remained reasonably high. Subsequently, Treadwell et al. conducted brief choice assessments (8-items) and reinforcer assessments with 4 clients. For each client, the assessments were completed in less than 2 hours, and effective reinforcers were identified.

In the investigations presented above, simple, arbitrary responses (e.g., sitting in chairs, standing in squares) were used as dependent measures to assess reinforcer effectiveness. However, the extent to which the use of such simple responses predicted reinforcer effectiveness when used for more complex and clinically relevant responses (e.g., in DRO schedules to reduce aberrant behavior) was unknown. Therefore, the extent to which stimulus preference assessments could be used to predict the effectiveness of stimuli when used in reinforcement-based procedures was examined in a series of investigations by Piazza and colleagues (Piazza, Fisher, Hanley, Hilker, & Derby, 1996; Piazza et al., 1998).

Piazza, Fisher, Hanley et al. (1996) used a modification of the single-item presentation method to predict the effectiveness of reinforcement-based procedures to treat the self-injurious behavior (SIB) of 2 clients. The modification consisted of a 30-s stimulus presentation, measurement of the client's interaction with the stimulus, and simultaneous measurement of the client's rate of SIB. Based on the results of the preference assessment, three categories of stimuli were identified: (a) high-preference stimuli associated with high levels of SIB (HP/HS), (b) high-preference stimuli associated with low levels of SIB (HP/LS), and (c) low-preference stimuli associated with low levels of SIB (LP/LS). As predicted by the preference assessment, the HP/HS stimuli resulted in increased SIB, and the LP/LS stimuli resulted in no changes in SIB when these stimuli were used in DRO schedules with 2 clients. However, the stimulus preference assessment failed to predict the effects of the HP/LS stimuli. That is, the HP/LS stimuli were demonstrated to function as reinforcers, but did not affect SIB when used in a DRO schedule. These results suggested that the stimulus preference assessment may be used to predict both the beneficial and negative side effects of stimuli when used in DRO schedules.

Subsequently, Piazza et al. (1998) used preference assessments to identify (a) stimuli that would compete with pica that was maintained by automatic reinforcement, and (b) the specific aspect of oral stimulation that functioned as automatic reinforcement. First, functional analyses of pica were conducted with 3 clients with life-threatening pica. The functional analyses indicated that the pica of all 3 clients was maintained, at least in part, by automatic reinforcement. Next, the stimulus preference assessment described by Piazza, Fisher, Hanley et al. (1996) was used to identify highly preferred stimuli that were associated with low levels of pica. These highly preferred stimuli were incorporated into reinforcement-based treatment packages to reduce successfully the pica of the 3 clients. Subsequent stimulus preference assessments were conducted for 2 of the clients in which items that produced different types of oral stimulation (e.g., hard vs. soft) were presented in order to evaluate the specific aspects of stimulation that were important in the maintenance of each clients' pica. The firmness of the item appeared to be the salient component of oral stimulation for both clients. Thus, Piazza et al. (1998) showed that the stimulus preference assessment could be used to (a) predict the effectiveness of reinforcement-based procedures to reduce pica and (b) identify specific sources of automatic reinforcement.

The aforementioned studies represent a growing body of literature on predicting and enhancing the effectiveness of reinforcers. The results of this line of research can be summarized as follows. First, a choice assessment is generally more effective than single-item presentation in predicting relative reinforcer effectiveness (Fisher et al., 1992). Second, caregiver report based on the RAISD structured interview improves the accuracy of reinforcer identification when compared to the use of items from a standard list (Fisher et al., 1996). Third, the choice assessment accurately predicts relative reinforcer value (Piazza, Fisher, Hagopian et al., 1996). In addition, the time efficiency of the choice assessment can be improved without sacrificing accuracy (Treadwell et al., 1994, May). Finally, stimulus preference assessments can be used to predict the effectiveness of reinforcement-based procedures to reduce aberrant behavior (Piazza, Fisher, Hanley et al., 1996; Piazza et al., 1998).

The technology for reinforcer identification has now reached a state where reinforcers can be identified very quickly, easily, and accurately. We should encourage caregivers (e.g., teachers, parents, and health-care workers) in our communities to assess reinforcers for individuals with autism on a regular basis and make reinforcer identification procedures a standard part of an individual's curriculum.

References

Cautela, J. R., & Kastenbaum, R. A. (1967). A reinforcement survey for use in therapy, training, and research. *Psychological Reports, 20,* 1115-1130.

Dattilo, J. (1986). Computerized assessment of preference for severely handicapped individuals. *Journal of Applied Behavior Analysis, 19,* 445-448.

Fisher, W. W., Piazza, C. C., Bowman, L. G., & Amari, A. (1996). Integrating caregiver report with a systematic choice assessment to enhance reinforcer identification. *American Journal on Mental Retardation, 101,* 15-25.

Fisher, W., Piazza, C. C., Bowman, L. G., Hagopian, L. P., Owens, J. C., & Slevin, I. (1992). A comparison of two approaches for identifying reinforcers for persons with severe to profound disabilities. *Journal of Applied Behavior Analysis, 25,* 491-498.

Green, C. W., Reid, D. H., Canipe, V. S., & Gardner, S. M. (1991). A comprehensive evaluation of reinforcer identification processes for persons with profound multiple handicaps. *Journal of Applied Behavior Analysis, 24,* 537-552.

Green, C. W., Reid, D. H., White, L. K., Halford, R. C., Brittain, D. P., & Gardner, S. M. (1988). Identifying reinforcers for persons with profound handicaps: Staff opinion versus systematic assessment of preferences. *Journal of Applied Behavior Analysis, 21,* 31-43.

Homme, L. E., Csanyi, A. P., Gonzales, M. A., & Rechs, J. R. (1969). *How to use contingency contracting in the classroom.* Champaign, IL: Research Press.

Pace, G. M., Ivancic, M. T., Edwards, G. L., Iwata, B. A., & Page, T. J. (1985). Assessment of stimulus preference and reinforcer value with profoundly retarded individuals. *Journal of Applied Behavior Analysis, 18,* 249-255.

Piazza, C. C., Fisher, W. W., Hagopian, L. P., Bowman, L. G., & Toole, L. (1996). Using a choice assessment to predict reinforcer effectiveness. *Journal of Applied Behavior Analysis, 29,* 1-9.

Piazza, C. C., Fisher, W. W., Hanley, G. P. , Hilker, K., & Derby, K. M. (1996). A preliminary procedure for predicting the positive and negative effects of reinforcement -based procedures. *Journal of Applied Behavior Analysis, 29,* 137-152.

Piazza, C. C., Fisher, W. W., Hanley, G. P., LeBanc, L. A., Worsdell, A. S., Lindaur, S. E. and Keeney, K. M. (1998). Treatment of pica through multiple analyses of its reinforcing functions. *Journal of Applied Behavior Analysis,* 31, 165-189.

Treadwell, K., Fisher, W., & Amari, A. (1994, May). *On the relative accuracy and efficiency of abbreviated reinforcer assessments.* Poster session presented at the 20th annual convention of the Association for Behavior Analysis, Atlanta, GA.

Wacker, D. P., Berg, W. K., Wiggins, B., Muldoon, M., & Cavanaugh, J. (1985). Evaluation of reinforcer preferences for profoundly handicapped students. *Journal of Applied Behavior Analysis, 18,* 173-178.

Discussion of Piazza, Fisher, Bowman, and Blakely-Smith

Developments in Reinforcer Identification

James E. Carr

University of Nevada

Reinforcer identification is one of the fastest growing areas in the applied behavior-analytic literature. Piazza, Fisher, Bowman, and Blakeley-Smith (this volume) provide a nice overview of the history of the area, highlighting important findings and directions for future research. The purpose of the current discussion is to briefly emphasize some of the findings reported by Piazza et al. (this volume) and identify themes that are particularly relevant for intervention with children diagnosed with autism.

Piazza et al. (this volume) discussed three studies that are especially important to the applied literature. First, Fisher, Piazza, Bowman, and Amari (1996) developed the Reinforcer Assessment for Individuals with Severe Disabilities (RAISD) in an effort to structure the stimulus recommendations made by caregivers. Previous research has shown that caregiver report is an unpredictable method of selecting potential reinforcers (e.g., Green et al., 1988). The RAISD is a promising alternative to unstructured methods of stimulus solicitation, with obvious practical implications. Second, Treadwell, Fisher, and Amari (1994) demonstrated that the paired-stimulus presentation method could be administered in a relatively brief period. Such a refinement should allow practitioners to administer the assessment more frequently and with greater ease. The work of Fisher et al. (1996) and Treadwell et al. represents a real sensitivity of researchers to clinical needs. Third, Piazza, Fisher, Hanley, Hilkes & Derby (1996) demonstrated that the rankings (or selection percentages) produced by a preference assessment might not provide enough information to select stimuli for reduction procedures. The authors demonstrated that stimuli that were associated with high levels of aberrant behavior during the preference assessment resulted in negligible behavior change, regardless of their selection percentages. I believe these data are among the most provocative in the literature and certainly warrant future replication and extension.

Along with the single-stimulus (Pace, Ivancic, Edwards, Iwata, & Page, 1985) and paired-stimulus (Fisher et al., 1992) presentation methods discussed by Piazza et al. (this volume), researchers have also evaluated the utility of the multiple-stimulus preference assessment (e.g., DeLeon & Iwata, 1996; Windsor, Piche, & Locke, 1994). In these assessments, all of the stimuli are simultaneously presented to the client. After the first selection is made, the client is instructed to select another until all of them have been chosen. DeLeon and Iwata demonstrated that this approach was generally as effective as the paired-stimulus methods and could be completed in less time. These findings represent an important movement in the area of reinforcer identification: the development of practitioner-oriented methods.

There have been only a few reinforcer identification studies that included children diagnosed with autism as participants (e.g., Mason, McGee, Farmer-Dougan, & Risley, 1989). Given the nature of typical intensive interventions with these children (i.e., frequent learning opportunities with programmed consequences), one might expect a more extensive literature. As with most behavioral interventions, paraprofessionals usually deliver the clinical services to children diagnosed with autism. Consequently, our methods must be efficient and user-friendly. As was noted by Piazza et al. (this volume), preference is a temporary phenomenon. Although some stimuli may be consistently preferred over time, many of them are not. Unfortunately, we have not yet developed a technology for identifying establishing operations that affect the momentary reinforcing values of our programmed consequences. However, one of the ways in which the issues of paraprofessional service delivery and inconsistent stimulus preference can be addressed is through the use of brief assessments that can be repeatedly administered over time.

Carr, Nicolson, and Higbee (1998) assessed the effectiveness of a brief multiple-stimulus presentation method for three children diagnosed with autism. The assessment consisted of three consecutive multiple-stimulus presentation sessions. After the stimulus preference assessment was conducted, high-, medium- and low-preference stimuli were selected for each participant. These stimuli were then administered contingently during acquisition programs in each of the participant's daily curriculum. The results of this reinforcement assessment showed that the degree of reinforcement effect achieved was positively correlated with stimulus preference. That is, highly preferred stimuli produced the strongest reinforcement effects. These results were similar to those reported by Piazza, Fisher, Hagopian, Bowman & Toole (1996). Although conceptually similar to other studies in this area, the work of Carr et al., Mason et al. (1989), and Treadwell et al. (1994) represents a move toward extending the literature into more practical areas, especially with respect to autism.

Many reinforcer identification studies have included target behaviors that have been referred to by some as "arbitrary." That is, they were not clinically relevant target behaviors, but were selected instead for their efficiency and sensitivity within experimental preparations. Although it is true that reinforcers often have response-specific effects, the criticisms against this approach are sometimes unfounded. Perhaps these studies can be best interpreted as technology development. In order to have a working technology that can be transferred into naturalistic environments, the methods often must be extensively studied in controlled situations. Once technology reaches the point at which it can be incorporated into naturalistic situations, the degree of inference associated with analogue research can then be greatly reduced. Some might argue that the time for more naturalistic research in this area is now, although there have already been several studies that incorporated clinically relevant target behaviors in their protocols (e.g., Carr et al., 1998; DeLeon & Iwata, 1996; Northup, George, Jones, Broussard, & Vollmer, 1996). It is likely that will see more of these types of studies in the immediate future.

Another important development in the area of reinforcer identification that is particularly relevant to children diagnosed with autism is the use of preference assessments to select stimuli for use in behavioral reduction programs. Many children diagnosed with autism exhibit stereotypic behaviors, some of which are maintained independent of the social environment. That is, the behaviors are reinforced by characteristics of their own emission. One common intervention for such behaviors is environmental enrichment. Recently, researchers have begun using stimulus preference assessments to select the "enriching" stimuli (e.g., Ringdahl, Vollmer, Marcus, & Roane, 1997). Data from these studies indicate that reductive procedures that incorporate stimuli selected using preference assessments are more effective than those that incorporate arbitrarily selected stimuli. These studies, including the work of Piazza, Fisher, Hanley et al. (1996), represent a major contribution of stimulus preference assessment to applied behavior analysis: the enhancement of decelerative interventions.

In conclusion, I commend Piazza et al. (this volume) for their succinct review of this important literature, as well as for their own research contributions. However, despite the tremendous expansion of this literature since the work of Pace et al. (1985), there remains much to do. Future research areas include the following: (a) the further development of efficient practitioner-oriented methods, (b) the delineation of schedule effects within preference assessments (e.g., DeLeon, Iwata, Goh, & Worsdell, 1997), (c) the integration of preference assessments with stimulus variation methods (e.g., Bowman, Piazza, Fisher, Hagopian, & Kogan, 1997), and (d) the extension of preference assessment technology to other clinical populations. Along with developments in areas such as functional assessment and intervention, research in the area of reinforcer identification represents real progress towards conceptually sound methods in applied behavior analysis.

References

Bowman, L. G., & Piazza, C. C., Fisher, W. W., Hagopian, L. P., & Kogan, J. S. (1997). Assessment of preference for varied versus constant reinforcers. *Journal of Applied Behavior Analysis, 30,* 451-458.

Carr, J. E., Nicolson, A. C., & Higbee, T. S. (1998). *Evaluation of a brief method for assessing stimulus preference with children diagnosed with autism.* Manuscript submitted for publication.

DeLeon, I. G., & Iwata, B. A. (1996). Evaluation of a multiple-stimulus presentation format for assessing reinforcer preferences. *Journal of Applied Behavior Analysis, 29,* 519-533.

DeLeon, I. G., Iwata, B. A., Goh, H., & Worsdell, A. S. (1997). Emergence of reinforcer preference as a function of schedule requirements and stimulus similarity. *Journal of Applied Behavior Analysis, 30,* 439-449.

Fisher, W. W., Piazza, C. C., Bowman, L. G., & Amari, A. (1996). Integrating caregiver report with a systematic choice assessment to enhance reinforcer identification. *American Journal on Mental Retardation, 101,* 15-25.

Fisher, W., Piazza, C. C., Bowman, L. G., Hagopian, L. P., Owens, J. C., & Slevin, I. (1992). A comparison of two approaches for identifying reinforcers for persons with severe and profound disabilities. *Journal of Applied Behavior Analysis, 25,* 491-498.

Green, C. W., Reid, D. H., White, L. K., Halford, R. C., Brittain, D. P., & Gardner, S. M. (1988). Identifying reinforcers for persons with profound handicaps: Staff opinion versus systematic assessments of preferences. *Journal of Applied Behavior Analysis, 21,* 31-43.

Mason, S. A., McGee, G. G., Farmer-Dougan, V., & Risley, T. R. (1989). A practical strategy for ongoing reinforcer assessment. *Journal of Applied Behavior Analysis, 22,* 171-179.

Northup, J., George, T., Jones, K., Broussard, C., & Vollmer, T. R. (1996). A comparison of reinforcer assessment methods: The utility of verbal and pictorial choice procedures. *Journal of Applied Behavior Analysis, 29,* 201-212.

Pace, G. M., Ivancic, M. T., Edwards, G. L., Iwata, B. A., & Page, T. A. (1985). Assessment of stimulus preference and reinforcer value with profoundly retarded individuals. *Journal of Applied Behavior Analysis, 18,* 249-255.

Piazza, C. C., Fisher, W. W., Hagopian, L. P., Bowman, L. G., & Toole, L. (1996). Using a choice assessment to predict reinforcer effectiveness. *Journal of Applied Behavior Analysis, 29,* 1-9.

Piazza, C. C., Fisher, W. W., Hanley, G. P., Hilker, K., & Derby, K. M. (1996). A preliminary procedure for predicting the positive and negative effects of reinforcement-based procedures. *Journal of Applied Behavior Analysis, 29,* 137-152.

Ringdahl, J. E., Vollmer, T. R., Marcus, B. A., & Roane, H. S. (1997). An analogue evaluation of environmental enrichment: The role of stimulus preference. *Journal of Applied Behavior Analysis, 30,* 203-216.

Treadwell, K., Fisher, W., & Amari, A. (1994, May). *On the relative accuracy and efficiency of abbreviated reinforcer assessments.* Poster session presented at the 20th annual convention of the Association for Behavior Analysis, Atlanta, GA.

Windsor, J., Piche, L. M., & Locke, P. A. (1994). Preference testing: A comparison of two presentation methods. *Research in Developmental Disabilities, 15,* 439-455.

Chapter 6

Interresponse Relations Among Aberrant Behaviors Displayed By Persons With Autism And Developmental Disabilities

**Wayne W. Fisher, Cathleen C. Piazza,
Cindy J. Alterson, and David E. Kuhn**
*Kennedy Krieger Institute
and Johns Hopkins University School of Medicine*

Functional Analysis

Most methods of assessing, diagnosing, and categorizing behavior focus on the physical characteristics or topography of the responses, and the extent to which certain response topographies co-occur. For example, if a child shows little or no facial expression, appears overly sensitive to sounds and touch, plays and arranges things in a rigid and specific manner, is more interested in inanimate objects than in people, and frequently displays repetitive motor movements, we might diagnose the child as having autism. This is an example of a structural method of categorizing behavior disorders, in which classification is according to the physical characteristics of the behavior.

An alternative, but not mutually exclusive method of diagnosing behavior disorders is one in which responses or symptoms are categorized according to their function, or the effect they have on the environment. Assessing and diagnosing behavior according to its function helps us better understand why the behavior occurs, and it allows us to prescribe specific treatments that are highly likely to be successful. For example, if an individual is referred for treatment of aggression, self-injurious behavior (SIB), and stereotypy and is categorized as having autism, that diagnosis does *not* help us prescribe a specific course of treatment. On the other hand, effective treatments can be readily identified if we accurately assess and diagnose the function(s) of each of the presenting problems. That is, if we can identify the purpose aggression serves, or the benefit the individual receives from the response, then there are specific actions we can take to decrease this aberrant behavior.

From a behavior-analytic perspective, SIB and other aberrant behaviors are viewed as operants, responses that operate on the environment and produce some effect or outcome. Skinner introduced the concept of the operant to help explain how the outcomes a response has produced in the past affect the likelihood that it will be repeated in the future. That is, responses that have operated on the environment and produced preferred or beneficial outcomes in the past are likely to be repeated in the future. Responses that have produced non-preferred or detrimental outcomes are *not* likely to be repeated. In this way, Skinner's notion of operant selection is analogous to Darwin's theory of natural selection. The characteristics of a species gradually evolve because those attributes that are successful and adaptive are selectively passed on to successive generations. Similarly, a given environment selects certain responses in an individual's behavioral repertoire over others, because some behaviors produce more successful, adaptive, or desirable outcomes.

One promising method for assessing and categorizing behavior according to its function is called functional analysis. Functional analysis is used to determine the extent to which the outcome or consequence of a behavior affects its probability. A fundamental characteristic of functional analysis that differentiates it from other assessments (e.g., interviews, standardized tests) is that the variables hypothesized to affect an individual's behavior are systematically manipulated in accordance with single-case, experimental design procedures. The systematic manipulation of the environmental events of interest provides a direct test of the extent to which these variables affect the target behavior.

The Development of Functional Analysis Methods

Early attempts at identifying and analyzing relations between environmental events and problem behavior generally involved the manipulation of a single environmental variable (Berkson & Mason, 1963; Carr, Newsom, & Binkoff, 1980; Lovaas & Simmons, 1969). Based in part on these prior investigations, three hypotheses regarding environmental influences for SIB were articulated by Carr (1977). One hypothesis was that destructive behavior was maintained by positive reinforcement in the form of contingent social attention. The second hypothesis was that destructive behavior was maintained by negative reinforcement in the form of escape from, or avoidance of, nonpreferred tasks or activities. The third hypothesis was that destructive behavior was a form of self-stimulation that provided its own automatic or intrinsic reinforcement. For example, visually impaired individuals with intact sensory pathways who display SIB often direct this response toward the eyes. This presumably occurs because eye poking or eye pressing stimulates the visual cortex, which may be highly reinforcing to someone who experiences very little visual stimulation.

The three hypotheses articulated by Carr (1977) are not mutually exclusive and any, all, or none of these environmental variables may influence the destructive behavior displayed by a particular individual. For example, one individual's aberrant behavior might be maintained by attention; another individual's behavior might be maintained by escape; and a third individual's behavior might be maintained by a combination of automatic reinforcement and attention. Thus, a valid assessment of how these environmental events influence destructive behavior would require the examination of each of these variables with individual clients. In 1982, Iwata and colleagues described a functional analysis procedure designed to examine simultaneously each of these three operant hypotheses for SIB (Iwata, Dorsey, Slifer, Bauman, & Richman, 1982/1994).

The functional analysis method originally developed and described by Iwata et al. (1982/1994) consisted of three test conditions (attention, demand, & alone) and one control condition (play). Each test condition was designed to test one of the hypotheses described by Carr (1977). In the attention condition, the client was given toys to play with while an adult was engaged in a separate activity (reading a magazine). If SIB occurred, the adult discontinued this activity and presented brief verbal and/or physical attention to the client (e.g., saying "Don't do that, you'll hurt yourself" and rubbing the site of the SIB). Thus, in this condition, the client was deprived of attention unless SIB occurred (i.e., the only time the client received adult attention was following SIB). This condition was designed to be an analogue of situations in which a caregiver is busy and not attending to the client. In such situations, most caregivers will normally stop what they are doing and attend to a client who engages in SIB. This condition was designed to test whether adult attention functions as reinforcement for SIB.

In the demand condition, the client was prompted to complete nonpreferred tasks. If SIB occurred, the therapist discontinued the task and provided the client with a short break. This condition was designed to be an analogue of situations in which caregivers are attempting to get the client to complete nonpreferred activities. In such situations, caregivers will often stop the activity when SIB occurs in order to give the client a chance to calm down. The purpose of this condition was to determine whether termination of nonpreferred tasks functioned as reinforcement for SIB.

During the alone condition, the client was placed in a room alone without toys or materials. This condition was designed to be an analogue of a sterile environment. Aberrant behavior that is maintained by the sensory stimulation it produces is most likely to occur in situations where there is nothing else to do (i.e., no competing sources of stimulation or reinforcement). This condition was designed to assess indirectly whether SIB produced its own (automatic) reinforcement.

In the play condition, the therapist and client played together with preferred toys or leisure materials. The therapist provided attention approximately once every 30 seconds after a 5-second period during which no SIB occurred. This condition was designed to be an analogue of an enriched environment, and served as a control for the test conditions.

The client was exposed to these four conditions during 15-minute sessions and each condition was conducted multiple times over several days (approximately 5 to 10 sessions per condition). The conditions were alternated randomly in accordance with a multielement design. Finally, the results were graphed and visually inspected to determine whether SIB occurred at differentially higher rates in one or more of the test conditions than in the control condition. Figure 1 shows an example

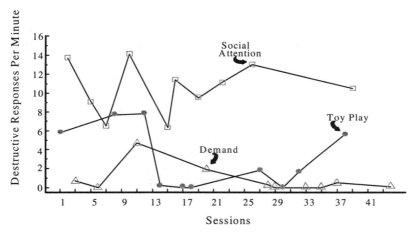

Figure 1.Rates of destructive responses during two test (demand, social attention) and one test (toy play) conditions. The conditions were alternated randomly throughout five to tensessions per day over several days.

of a functional analysis graph for an individual who displayed aberrant behavior maintained by attention.

The Impact of Functional Analysis Methods

Over the last 15 years, this clinical and research technology called functional analysis has been developed and refined systematically to identify and assess how the environmental and social consequences produced by aberrant behavior affect the development and maintenance of these problems. The seminal work on functional analysis methods by Iwata and colleagues has dramatically altered how we analyze and treat SIB and other aberrant behaviors displayed by individuals with autism and other developmental disabilities. One significant advancement has been the advent of experimental-epidemiological studies designed to evaluate operant hypotheses about the maintenance of problem behavior (e.g., Derby et al., 1992; Iwata, Pace, Dorsey et al., 1994). For example, Iwata, Pace, Dorsey et al. conducted an epidemiological investigation of SIB, which included the results of 152 experimental functional analyses. Interestingly, the operant hypotheses described by Carr (1977) accounted for the vast majority of the cases of SIB. In 23% of the cases, SIB was maintained by attention. In 35.4% of the cases, SIB was maintained by escape. Finally, in 25.7% of the cases, the results suggested that SIB was maintained by automatic reinforcement.

A second significant advancement that has resulted from functional analysis research has been the refinement of treatment procedures like extinction, differential reinforcement, and punishment. For example, an extinction procedure for a response maintained by negative reinforcement looks quite different from an extinction procedure for a response maintained by attention (cf. Iwata, Pace, Cowdery, & Miltenberger, 1994). Similarly, differential reinforcement procedures that use reinforcers identified through a functional analysis remove the specific establishing operation for aberrant behavior, and therefore may be more effective than other differential reinforcement interventions (Fisher, Lindauer, Alterson, & Thompson, 1998).

A third significant advancement that has resulted from functional analysis research has been the rapid development of novel and effective treatment strategies for aberrant behavior (e.g., Bowman, Fisher, Thompson, & Piazza, 1997; Chapman, Fisher, Piazza, & Kurtz, 1993; Dunlap, Kern-Dunlap, Clarke, & Robbins, 1991; Horner, Day, Sprague, O'Brien, & Heathfield, 1991; Kennedy & Souza, 1995; Mace & Belfiore, 1990; Pace, Iwata, Cowdery, Andree, & McIntyre, 1993; Touchette, MacDonald, & Langer, 1985; Vollmer, Iwata, Zarcone, Smith, & Mazaleski, 1993). In general, treatments based on the function or purpose of aberrant behavior are often aimed at removing the reinforcement responsible for the behavior's maintenance (teaching the autistic child that outbursts of aggression no longer produce social isolation). In addition, the individual is often taught alternative, appropriate behaviors that can produce the same environmental or social benefit (teaching appropriate ways to request periods of solitude). Finally, procedures are often included that help the individual learn to tolerate better the situations that lead to aberrant behavior (teaching a child with autism to more easily endure social activities).

Interresponse Relations

The functional analysis method developed by Iwata et al. (1982/1994) was originally designed for individuals with mental retardation who exhibited severe SIB. Over the past 15 years, these basic procedures have been adapted and used with a variety of disorders and target behaviors (e.g., Chapman et al., 1993; Cooper, Wacker, Sasso, Reimers, & Donn, 1990; Dunlap et al., 1991; Fisher et al., 1993). Over the past several years, we have attempted to refine functional analysis methods in order to analyze and treat multiple aberrant responses that are functionally related to one another. Our interest in this topic began with the observation (made by many colleagues) that SIB and self-restraint often co-occur. That is, self-restraint occurs almost exclusively among individuals who display SIB. Although this relation between self-restraint and SIB may be the most striking example of two correlated problem behaviors, it is actually the rule, rather than the exception, that individuals who exhibit one aberrant response (e.g., aggression) often display other aberrant responses as well (e.g., SIB; Griffin, Williams, Stark, Altmeyer, & Mason, 1986; Maurice & Trudel, 1982; Powell, Bodfish, Parker, Crawford, & Lewis, 1996; Sigafoos, Elkins, Kerr, & Attwood, 1994).

Explanations regarding the apparent co-occurrence of aberrant behaviors remain somewhat tentative, perhaps because most investigations on how aberrant behaviors relate to one another have employed correlational, rather than experimental methods (e.g., Aman, Singh, Stewart, & Field, 1985; Griffin et al., 1986). Functional analysis methods can provide more direct evaluations of operant hypotheses about relations between co-occurring aberrant responses. Before discussing the applied research on this topic, it may be helpful first to review briefly the operant principles pertaining to interresponse relations derived from basic research.

Basic Research and Principles on Interresponse Relations

Responses as reinforcement. The idea that a response can function as a reinforcer was discussed many years ago by Sheffield and colleagues (e.g. Sheffield, Roby, & Campbell, 1954), who formulated the consummatory-response theory. Essentially, this theory stated that consummatory behaviors, such as eating and drinking, were the critical elements that make certain tangible items, such as food and drink, effective reinforcers. Viewed from this perspective, it is the act of eating and drinking, rather than the food or drink, that is reinforcing. This theory posited that consummatory behaviors were unique in that they could function as effective reinforcers, whereas other behaviors generally could not. David Premack challenged this assumption by suggesting that just about any operant response could function as reinforcement, or be reinforced by another response, depending on the circumstances of the situation (Premack, 1965).

Premack (1965) argued that the critical variable that determined the reinforcing potential of a response was its probability of occurrence relative to the probability of the target response. That is, the Premack principle states that a response with a higher probability of occurrence can function as reinforcement for another response with a lower probability of occurrence. According to the Premack principle, higher probability responses can reinforce lower probability responses, but not vice versa. The way in which Premack determined the relative probabilities of behaviors was to allow the participant access to all of the potential target and reinforcement responses concurrently, and then to measure the proportion of time engaged in each response. In experiments on this topic, the reinforced behavior is often called the "instrumental response," and the behavior that is presented as reinforcement is often called the "contingent response." Premack argued that a response that occurred for a greater proportion of the free-operant baseline would subsequently function as an effective "contingent response" for an "instrumental response" that occurred less during the baseline.

In one of his studies, Premack (1971) allowed young children free access to two responses: eating candy and playing pinball. In this baseline, some of the children spent more time eating candy, whereas others spent more time playing pinball. When the opportunity to engage in eating candy was made contingent upon the occurrences of playing pinball, only the children who spent more time eating in the baseline condition showed a reinforcement effect (i.e., increased the rate of playing from baseline). When the opportunity to engage in playing pinball was made contingent upon occurrences of eating candy, only the children who spent more time playing in the baseline condition increased the rate of eating. These results clearly showed that both eating and playing pinball could function as reinforcement, although the former was a consummatory response and the latter was not. The results also showed that the relative probabilities of these two responses (eating and playing pinball) predicted when each one would and would not function as reinforcement for the other.

Contrary to the Premack principle, a number of investigations have shown that lower probability responses can function as reinforcement for higher probability responses if certain conditions are met (e.g., Eisenberger, Karpman, & Trattner, 1967). In addition, higher probability responses sometimes fail to function as reinforcers for lower probability responses (e.g., Konarski, Johnson, Crowell, & Whitman, 1980). Response deprivation theory, a refinement of the Premack principle, was developed to explain these situations and better predict the reinforcing effects of responses (Timberlake & Allison, 1974). According to this theory, a contingent response will function as reinforcement if it occurs at some (non-zero) level during a free-operant baseline, and the contingency in effect produces "response deprivation" (i.e., the individual has decreased access to this "contingent" response unless the target response increases). Under these conditions, lower probability responses can function as reinforcement for higher probability responses (Konarski, 1987).

Automatic reinforcement and interresponse relations. With both the Premack principle and response deprivation theory, the reinforcing effects of responses are predicted based on how often the behaviors occur during a free-operant baseline. One response can function as reinforcement for another response if the contingency restricts access to the contingent response below its free-operant level. However, why do these responses occur at all during free-operant baselines, and why do they function as reinforcement for other responses? Well, if the response is an operant, and it occurs at a relatively high, free-operant level, then presumably the response produces some form of desirable stimulation.

Although is not often discussed in relation to the reinforcement effects of responses, the concept of automatic reinforcement may be relevant to many interresponse relations. Automatic reinforcement is a term that refers to operant mechanisms hypothesized to be responsible for the maintenance of behaviors that persist in the absence of social contingencies (Skinner, 1953; Vaughn & Michael, 1982; Vollmer, 1994). That is, some responses may produce their own reinforcement automatically. For example, loosening one's tie may be automatically reinforced by the discomfort it relieves. Similarly, responses that persist during free-operant baselines (e.g., eating, playing pinball) may do so because they produce some form of reinforcing stimulation automatically. As previously mentioned, a variety of aberrant responses (e.g., pica, stereotypies) persist in the absence of social contingencies (i.e., have high free-operant levels) and therefore appear to be maintained by automatic reinforcement. Thus, automatically-maintained aberrant responses may function as effective reinforcers when their access is restricted (causing response deprivation) and presented contingent upon some other, "instrumental" response. In fact, a number of studies have shown that contingent access to stereotypic behavior can be used as reinforcement for appropriate target responses (e.g., compliance; Charlop, Kurtz, & Casey, 1990; Sugai & White, 1986).

Other basic research on interresponse relations. Although much of the basic research on interresponse relations has focussed on how behaviors may function as reinforcement for one other, a response may influence the probability of another response through other operant mechanisms as well. That is, responses often precede, occur in place of, or follow one another. Thus, one response may influence the probability of another response by acting on any of the components of the operant, three-term contingency (antecedent-behavior-consequence). For example, when lever pressing is maintained on a differential reinforcement of low rate schedule, rats will develop collateral responses that apparently function as discriminative stimuli that allow them to track more accurately the passage of time (e.g., Laties, Weiss, & Weiss, 1969). One response may also exert stimulus control by acting as an establishing operation and altering motivation for another response. For example, eating salty food generally increases the reinforcement value of drinking (Michael, 1993). In addition, one response may develop and maintain because it increases the probability of reinforcement for another response. For example, Polson and Parsons (1994) showed that three of four college students quickly learned to press the left key of a computer mouse when it increased the probability of reinforcement for presses made on the right key. Finally, others have shown that arranging reinforcement contingencies for what people say they will do may sometimes influence their actions more than when their actions are directly reinforced (cf. Catania, Mathews, & Shimoff, 1982).

Analysis and Treatment of Functionally-Related Aberrant Responses

Two aberrant responses may co-occur for a variety of reasons. Some of the reasons may be related to one or more of the operant mechanisms described above, whereas others may not. For example, children with autism often display pronomial reversals (e.g., saying "You" when they mean "I") and stereotypic hand flapping. Although these two responses often co-occur, it is highly doubtful that this is due to operant mechanisms. However, some aberrant behaviors are connected through operant mechanisms, and we shall now turn our attention to these responses and the ways in which they relate to one another.

Members of a common operant class. Two aberrant responses are functionally related when the function of one response topography is in some way tied to or affected by the presence or absence of the other response. Perhaps the simplest way in which two or more topographically distinct aberrant responses may be functionally related is when they are members of the same operant class (i.e., maintained by the same reinforcer). Smith, Iwata, Vollmer, and Pace (1992) conducted a functional analysis of SIB showing that a response was maintained by escape from nonpreferred tasks, and suggested that self-restraint was maintained by the same reinforcement. Similarly, Derby, Fisher, and Piazza (1996) alternately delivered attention noncontingently or contingent on either the SIB or self-restraint of a girl with tuberous sclerosis and profound mental retardation. This analysis showed that both SIB and self-restraint were maintained by contingent attention. Finally, Lalli, Mace,

Wohn, and Livezy (1995) conducted a series of analyses showing that three responses (screaming, aggression, and SIB) were hierarchical members of the same response class, and all were maintained by escape. When demands were presented, the individual screamed. If this did not produce escape, screaming was replaced by aggression. If neither screaming nor aggression produced escape, SIB occurred. These case studies illustrate how topographically distinct responses may sometimes be functionally related, because each one produces the same reinforcement. Nevertheless, case studies do *not* specify how common it is for topographically distinct responses to be related in this manner.

Derby et al. (1998) reviewed a series of 50 functional analyses to assess how often topographically different responses (e.g., aggression, SIB) belonged either to the same or different operant classes. In 42% of the cases (n = 21), clear operant functions were identified for 2 or more response topographies (e.g., aggression, pica, SIB). Surprisingly, within this subset of 21 cases, it was rare for all of a client's topographies to belong to the same response class (n = 3 or 14% of the cases). More often (n = 11 or 52% of the cases), each topographically distinct response belonged to a separate operant class. Finally, in one third of the cases (n = 7), two topographies belonged to one response class (e.g., SIB and aggression maintained by escape) and one or more other topographies had a different function (e.g., property destruction maintained by attention). These results suggest that the simplest operant explanation as to why topographically different aberrant responses may be correlated (i.e., that they belong to the same operant class) applies to a small minority of cases. Therefore, it may be useful for behavior analysts to examine other ways in which topographically different aberrant responses may be functionally related.

One response alters motivation for another one. Responses are often preceded and followed by other responses. Premack pointed out that a response that follows another one may function as reinforcement for the preceding response. However, it is also the case that a response that precedes another one may exert stimulus control over the subsequent response.

Michael (1993) argued that it may be important to distinguish between two types of antecedent stimuli that exert control over operant behavior: those that signal the availability of reinforcement (discriminative stimuli), and those that alter motivation (establishing operations). Establishing operations affect operant responding by temporarily altering the reinforcing effectiveness of consequent stimuli. The clearest examples of establishing operations are satiation and deprivation. Recent work on antecedent influences on problem behavior has shown that establishing operations can dramatically alter the probability of aberrant behavior (see Smith & Iwata, 1997, for a review). For example, a number of investigations have shown or suggested that a variety of antecedent events (e.g., deprivation of food or sleep, cancellation of preferred events) can evoke aberrant responses or alter the reinforcing effectiveness of various consequences (e.g., escape, tangible items; Horner, Day, & Day, 1997; Kennedy & Meyer, 1996; O'Reilly, 1995; Wacker et al., 1996). Conversely, the delivery of preferred stimuli or escape on a fixed-time schedule, sometimes referred to as "noncontingent" reinforcement, can decrease aberrant responses maintained by attention, tangible items, or escape (e.g., Hagopian, Fisher, & Legacy, 1994; Vollmer, Marcus, & Ringdahl, 1995; Vollmer, Ringdahl, Roane, & Marcus, 1997).

Given that aberrant responses often occur in close temporal proximity (i.e., one following another), it seems reasonable to hypothesize that one response topography may sometimes exert stimulus control over another one. For example, physical exercise has been shown to decrease aberrant behaviors, such as aggression, SIB, and stereotypies, even though the contingencies for these behaviors remained unchanged (e.g., Allison, Basile, & MacDonald, 1991; Baumeister & MacLean, 1984). One explanation of the effects of antecedent exercise is that this activity (i.e., response) acts as an establishing operation, and lowers the efficacy of the reinforcers that maintain aberrant behavior (Smith & Iwata, 1997). Although it has not been reported, it is also possible that exercise could potentially increase the effectiveness of the reinforcers that maintain aberrant behavior. For example, activities that produce fatigue could potentially increase the effectiveness of escape as reinforcement for aberrant behavior just as sleep deprivation does (e.g., Horner et al., 1997). Finally, the occurrence of one aberrant behavior maintained by automatic reinforcement (e.g., stereotypy) could momentarily decrease the effectiveness of attention as reinforcement for another aberrant response (e.g., attention-maintained aggression). A recent investigation by Thompson, Fisher, Piazza, and Kuhn (in press) provides a nice illustration of how one response may alter the effectiveness of reinforcement for another response.

Thompson et al. (in press) used direct and indirect functional analyses to assess and treat multiple topographies of aggression that belonged to separate operant classes in a young boy (Ernie) with pervasive developmental disorder (PDD) and mental retardation. A functional analysis of aggression using the methods described by Iwata et al. (1982/1994) produced inconclusive results. Next, descriptive assessments were conducted and used to generate hypotheses about the functions of the different topographies of aggression. These assessments led to the hypotheses that: (a) one topography of aggression, chin grinding (firmly pressing and grinding his chin against the skin and bones of others), was maintained by automatic reinforcement; and (b) the other topographies (e.g., hitting, kicking) were maintained by attention. A second, more specific functional analysis was then designed to test these hypotheses. In this analysis, attention was delivered either noncontingently, contingent on all forms of aggression, or contingent on other aggression (e.g., hitting, kicking, but not chin grinding).

The results of this second functional analysis are shown in the top (chin grinding) and bottom (other aggression) panels of Figure 2. As can be seen, chin grinding persisted across all conditions regardless of whether it produced attention or not, thus supporting the hypothesis that it was maintained by automatic reinforcement. By contrast, other aggression occurred at near-zero levels except when it was the only way for Ernie to obtain attention (i.e., during the CA[Other] condition).

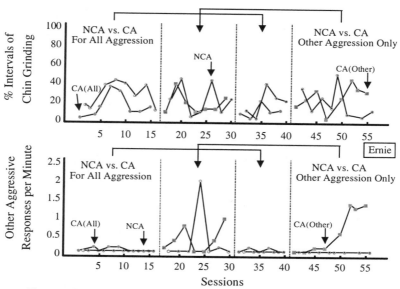

Figure 2. Represents the results of the second functional analysis with Ernie.

These results illustrate how a contingency for one response may have no effect on that behavior, but may decrease another response. The delivery of attention for chin grinding did not affect this response, presumably because it was maintained by automatic reinforcement (chin stimulation). However, the contingency for chin grinding decreased the probability of other aggression to near-zero levels, even though this latter response continued to produce attention. Thus, the delivery of attention contingent on chin grinding was similar to "free" or "noncontingent" reinforcement (e.g., Hagopian et al., 1994). Ernie was already engaging in chin grinding due to the automatic reinforcement it produced. Thus, the attention delivered contingent on this response amounted to a bonus, because he didn't expend any extra energy to get the attention. The delivery of the "bonus" reinforcement lowered Ernie's motivation to engage in other aggression. That is, it functioned as an establishing operation (Michael, 1993). Subsequent analyses showed that a treatment designed for attention-maintained behavior lowered other aggression, but not chin grinding. Chin grinding was reduced to clinically acceptable levels only when the presumed response-reinforcer relation was discontinued (through blocking), and an alternative form of chin stimulation was provided to Ernie. These treatment evaluation results confirmed that the two behaviors were members of separate operant classes.

One response alters reinforcement probability for another one. Polson and Parsons (1994) showed how one response might be reinforced by increasing the probability of reinforcement for another response. A similar relation may sometimes develop between mands and aberrant behavior. Skinner (1957) defined a mand as an operant that specifies its reinforcer (e.g., "Please give me a drink"). However, a mand does not guarantee that the specified reinforcer will be delivered. Skinner suggested that an individual can increase the probability that another individual will reinforce a mand through either positive reinforcement (e.g., saying "Thank you") or negative reinforcement (e.g., following through on the threat, "Give me a drink or else!"). Bowman et al. (1997) showed that mands and destructive behavior are occasionally related in this way.

The participants in the Bowman et al. (1997) investigation seemed to "boss their parents around." That is, they displayed a high rate of mands, many of which were unreasonable (e.g., asking family members to sit on each other's laps during meals). The participants displayed destructive behavior primarily when their mands did not produce reinforcement (i.e., when their parents did not comply with the mands or requests). The parents could avoid this destructive behavior by reinforcing all or almost all of the participant's mands, which they did (even the unreasonable ones). Thus, mands functioned to produce a wide variety of requested reinforcers, and the

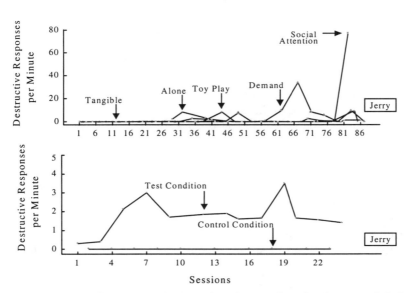

Figure 3. The top panel represents a functional analysis conducted with Jerry and the bottom panel a mand analysis.

function of destructive behavior was to increase the likelihood that all or almost all requests would produce reinforcement.

Figure 3 shows the results of two analyses conducted with one of the participants in the Bowman et al. (1997) investigation. Jerry was a 12-year-old boy with mild to moderate mental retardation, PDD, attention deficit-hyperactivity disorder, and a seizure disorder. The top panel shows the results of a functional analysis conducted using the methods described by Iwata et al. (1982/1994), which, as can be seen, produced inconclusive results. The bottom panel shows the results of an analysis (called the mand analysis) based on the hypothesis that the function of destructive behavior was to increase the probability that mands would produce the reinforcers they specified. In the control condition, the therapist reinforced all mands, and destructive behavior produced no differential consequences. In the test condition, the therapist discontinued reinforcement of mands at the start of the

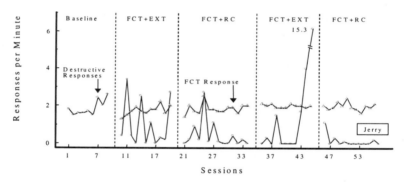

Figure 4. Represents treatment conditions and results for Jerry.

session and resumed compliance with mands for 30 seconds contingent on destructive behavior. As can be seen, destructive behavior occurred exclusively in this latter condition, where its function was to increase reinforcement for mands.

Figure 4 shows the results of the treatment evaluation conducted with Jerry in the Bowman et al. (1997) investigation. During baseline, destructive behavior functioned to increase reinforcement for mands (it was identical to the test condition of the mand analysis). During functional communication training with extinction (FCT + EXT), an appropriate communication response (the statement, "Please play by my rules") resulted in reinforcement of Jerry's mands for 30 seconds, and destructive behavior produced no consequence (i.e., extinction). As can be seen, this treatment reduced, but did not eliminate, destructive behavior. We then added a response cost procedure in which the therapist terminated reinforcement of mands contingent on destructive behavior. The combination of differential reinforcement of an alternative communication response and the response cost contingency reduced destructive behavior to near-zero levels. Over time, fading and discrimination training procedures were used to teach Jerry that some mands were inappropriate and would not produce reinforcement, and that even appropriate mands would not be reinforced all of the time (e.g., during work activities).

The relation between mands and destructive behavior may develop in some individuals because the combination of these two responses allows them efficiently and effectively to access a wide array of reinforcers. It is clear that most individuals prefer different reinforcers at different points in time. Mands specify the reinforcers that are most preferred at various points in time and destructive behavior increases the likelihood that the requested activities or objects are delivered.

One response functions as reinforcement for another. As the basic research on interresponse relations has shown, one (contingent) response can function as reinforcement for another (instrumental) response if the contingency between the two responses restricts access to the contingent response below its free-operant level (Timberlake & Allison, 1974). As mentioned above, the contingent response is usually the more probable response, but it doesn't have to be.

Fisher, Adelinis, Thompson, Worsdell, and Zarcone (in press) suggested that aberrant responses displayed by individuals with autism and mental retardation, such as SIB, pica, rituals, and stereotypies, often persist in the absence of social contingencies, and are presumably maintained by automatic reinforcement. Parents and teachers often interrupt these responses during the course of a normal day (e.g., through blocking or instructing the child to do an incompatible activity). Interrupting an automatically maintained response is analogous to an extinction procedure (or Type II punishment), because the individual is deprived of positive reinforcement. It is technically not extinction, because the response does not occur in the absence of reinforcement. Nevertheless, interrupting an automatically maintained response effectively terminates its reinforcer, which may increase the probability that another response will emerge, one typically evoked by reinforcement deprivation (e.g., tantrums, aggression, SIB). If a parent or teacher is blocking an aberrant response (e.g., a ritual) and this produces a more severe aberrant response (e.g., SIB), they are likely to terminate the blocking procedure. Termination of the blocking procedure may allow the individual to resume the automatically maintained response (e.g., stereotypies). Because the automatically maintained response is generally a preferred activity, its resumption may, in turn, function as reinforcement for the evoked responses (e.g., aggression or SIB).

Smith, Lerman, and Iwata (1996) recently published a case report showing this type of relation between SIB and self-restraint. They conducted an analysis with a blind woman with profound mental retardation showing that SIB, a relatively lower probability response, was maintained by contingent access to self-restraint, a relatively higher probability response. Contingencies like these, between two aberrant responses, may be most likely to develop in the natural environment among individuals who frequently display automatically maintained aberrant behaviors, and who react strongly when these responses are interrupted. For example, children with autism frequently display a variety of inflexible routines, rituals, and stereotypies.

In addition, these responses often appear to persist in the absence of social contingencies, suggesting that they may be maintained by automatic reinforcement. Moreover, children with autism often strongly react when their routines are changed unexpectedly or their rituals or stereotypies are interrupted. For these reasons, we have recently conducted analyses with children diagnosed with autism to determine whether they sometimes display aggression, property destruction, or SIB when their rituals or stereotypies are interrupted, and whether contingent access to these latter behaviors functions as reinforcement for the former ones.

We recently completed a series of analyses with a 5-year-old boy with autism and mental retardation named Mike (Fisher, 1998). First, a functional analysis was conducted using the methods described by Iwata et al. (1982/1994). However, Mike rarely displayed aggression during this analysis. We then conducted descriptive assessments that suggested three potential functions of aggression, namely, that aggression was maintained by: (a) negative reinforcement in the form of escape from demands, (b) negative reinforcement in the form of escape from social interaction, or (c) positive reinforcement in the form of contingent access to stereotypies. A series of analyses was then conducted that clearly showed that termination of demands and social interaction functioned as reinforcement only when they interfered with or interrupted Mike's stereotypy. That is, demands and social interaction that interrupted stereotypies evoked aggression, and termination of those activities allowed Mike to resume stereotypy. Thus, aggression was maintained by positive reinforcement (access to a preferred activity, stereotypy) and not by escape from demands or social interaction.

Termination of "don't" requests and aberrant behavior. Parents often tell their children to terminate undesirable behaviors (e.g., "stop jumping on the bed"). In the behavioral literature, this type of demand has been referred to as a "don't" request (Neef, Shafer, Egel, Cataldo, & Parrish, 1983). "Don't" requests issued to individuals with autism may often be designed to interrupt automatically-maintained aberrant responses (e.g., "stop spinning"). When a "don't" request effectively terminates an automatically maintained behavior, it may produce response deprivation (i.e., reinforcement deprivation) and evoke other aberrant responses. These evoked responses (e.g., aggression, SIB) may be reinforced if they result in termination of the "don't" request and allow the individual to resume the automatically maintained aberrant behavior. Fisher et al. (in press) conducted a series of analyses showing how this can occur.

One of the participants in the Fisher et al. (in press) investigation was Tina, an adolescent girl with PDD, bipolar disorder, severe mental retardation, and a seizure disorder. First, a functional analysis of aggression was conducted using the procedures described by Iwata et al. (1982/1994). The results of this analysis were inconclusive. Therefore, we then conducted a series of descriptive assessments to generate hypotheses regarding potential idiosyncratic functions of aggression. Two such hypotheses were generated. One hypothesis was that demands involving gross-motor activity evoked destructive behavior. The second hypothesis was that instructional demands evoked problem behavior primarily when they interrupted an ongoing high probability activity (e.g., a "don't" request that interrupted stereotypic pacing). We then conducted an experimental analysis with two test conditions and one control condition to examine these specific hypotheses.

In one of the test conditions, "don't" requests were issued approximately once every 30 to 60 seconds. These requests interrupted an ongoing high probability activity (i.e., whatever Tina was doing at the time). If Tina displayed aggression following the "don't" request, the request was terminated for 30 seconds and she was allowed to resume the high probability activity. In the matched "do" request condition, requests were issued that involved levels of gross-motor activity similar to the level required in the "don't" request condition. If Tina displayed aggression, the demand was terminated for 30 seconds. In the control condition, no requests were presented and Tina was allowed to choose from a variety of free-operant responses. During this analysis, Tina displayed high rates of aggression in the "don't" request condition, and near-zero rates in the other two conditions. Furthermore, when termination of "don't" requests was contingent only on an appropriate alternative response during treatment with FCT and extinction, aggression decreased to near-zero levels and was replaced by appropriate communication.

The results presented by Fisher et al. (in press) suggest that aberrant behavior evoked by demands may sometimes be maintained by positive reinforcement rather than escape. That is, the activity that is interrupted by the request may be one that produces automatic, positive reinforcement. The demand interrupts this activity, thus producing response deprivation, which may evoke aggression. Allowing the individual to resume the preferred activity (which may often be a stereotypic response) contingent on aggression may function as reinforcement for this latter response. Tina was first taught to request termination of "don't" requests through an appropriate mand, and over time, she was gradually exposed to situations in which compliance with "don't" requests was mandatory.

Aberrant response chains maintained by automatic reinforcement. In many of the cases described above, stereotypic or ritualistic behavior functioned as reinforcement for other aberrant behaviors (e.g., aggression), and the contingency between these two responses was socially mediated. That is, another individual (e.g., a parent) interrupted the stereotypic or ritualistic behavior, and discontinued the interruption procedure contingent on aggression, SIB, or property destruction. However, two responses can form a response chain that is automatically reinforced by its terminal outcome. For example, foraging is viewed as a complex response chain maintained by its terminal link (i.e., consumption of food; Catania, 1998). Earlier components of the response chain (e.g., traveling to another feeding location, searching for food) occur primarily when they are necessary for producing the terminal outcome (e.g., when food becomes scarce in the initial location). Fisher et al. (1998) showed how two topographically-different aberrant responses displayed by children with autism or PDD may form an analogous response chain maintained by automatic reinforcement.

The two participants in the Fisher et al. (1998) study displayed property destruction (breaking objects, tearing or cutting materials, such as curtains) and stereotypic responses involving the same items (tapping the broken objects, string play with the torn material). We hypothesized that the two aberrant responses formed a response chain (i.e., property destruction followed by stereotypy) that was automatically maintained by its terminal outcome (i.e., the sensory stimulation produced by stereotypy). That is, stereotypy presumably occurred because it produced preferred sensory stimulation. Stereotypy was often preceded by property destruction, which provided the participants with preferred materials with which to engage in stereotypy and produce sensory stimulation.

The results of the analysis conducted with one of the participants in the Fisher et al. (1998) investigation may help to illustrate how this type of interresponse relation may develop. During baseline, Milo was alone in a room baited with plastic item similar to the objects he destroyed at home. The test condition, noncontingent destruction (NCD), was identical to baseline except that the room also contained previously destroyed objects (i.e., ones Milo destroyed in a previous session). As expected, stereotypy persisted across all phases. However, the availability of previously destroyed materials reduced property destruction by more than one half when it was initially introduced and to zero during the last four sessions of the second NCD phase. In addition, within-session analyses of the baseline conditions showed that property destruction was much more probable during the first minute of the session, whereas stereotypy was more probable thereafter, which further supported the response-chain hypothesis.

These results support the hypothesis that property destruction and stereotypy were members of a response chain that was maintained by automatic reinforcement. The fact that NCD reduced property destruction supports our hypothesis that it was maintained by the terminal consequence (i.e., the sensory reinforcement automatically produced by stereotypy). If property destruction produced a reinforcing consequence in and of itself (e.g., the tactile feel or sound of breaking objects), then the presence of previously destroyed items during NCD should not have reduced this response. However, if its function was to produce preferred materials for stereotypy, property destruction became unnecessary when such materials were noncontingently available during NCD. That is, property destruction was necessary only when no preferred (i.e., broken) materials were available with which to produce the sensory consequences of stereotypy (e.g., just as moving to a new location is a necessary component of foraging only when food becomes scarce).

Concluding Comments

Both appropriate and aberrant responses are often preceded and followed by other responses. The basic research literature on interresponse relations has identified a variety of operant mechanisms through which one response can be correlated with, or linked to, another one. The applied investigations reviewed above suggest that aberrant behaviors may sometimes be related to one another through these same operations. Two aberrant responses may be correlated because they belong to the same operant class or because one response affects the function of another response. One response may exert stimulus control over a second one by acting as an establishing operation and reducing the reinforcing effectiveness of the second response (e.g., Thompson et al., in press). In addition, an aberrant response may maintain because it increases the probability of reinforcement of another response, such as mands (e.g., Bowman et al., 1997). Finally, an aberrant response that persists in the absence of social contingencies may produce its own (automatic) reinforcement. Aberrant responses that produce reinforcement automatically (e.g., stereotypies, rituals, self-restraint, pica) may also function as reinforcement for other aberrant responses (e.g., aggression).

The model we have proposed regarding how automatically maintained aberrant responses (e.g., stereotypy, rituals) can function as reinforcement for destructive behavior (e.g., aggression, SIB, property destruction) may be particularly relevant to individuals with autism. Individuals with autism or PDD spend a great deal of time engaging in ritualistic and stereotypic responses, and these responses may often be maintained by automatic reinforcement. Parent, teachers, and other caregivers sometimes interrupt these rituals or stereotypies by issuing "don't" requests (e.g., "Stop that") or by physically blocking the responses. Interrupting autistic rituals and stereotypies may result in response deprivation, which, in turn, may evoke other aberrant responses (e.g., aggression, SIB). Given the strong emotional reactions children with autism sometimes display when their routines are changed or their rituals are interrupted, it is not difficult to envision how this second set of aberrant behaviors (e.g., aggression) might emerge. If parents, teachers, or other caregivers terminate their interruption procedures when these destructive behaviors occur, individuals with autism may then resume their preferred rituals or stereotypies, thus reinforcing the destructive behavior.

We began this chapter by discussing how environments select certain responses in an individual's behavioral repertoire over others. Responses that produce more desirable outcomes tend to be selected over those that produce less or undesirable outcomes. Functional analysis methods provide us with a technology for analyzing and understanding how the outcomes produced by aberrant responses contribute to their maintenance. We have discussed some recent extensions of the functional analysis method specifically designed to analyze interresponse relations. In some of these cases, two responses combined to produce an outcome that was not possible through either response alone. For example, the combination of mands supported by destructive behavior (e.g., "Do as I say or I'll hit myself") allowed the participants of the Bowman et al. (1997) investigation to specify and obtain a wide variety of reinforcers that could *not* have been fully accessed by either response alone. Similarly, the combination of property destruction and stereotypy allowed the participants in the Fisher et al. (1998) investigation to produce sensory consequences that were not obtainable by either response independently. Ascertaining how different behaviors may combine to produce desirable outcomes through extensions of functional analysis methodology should greatly improve our understanding of and ability to treat aberrant behavior displayed by persons with autism and other developmental disabilities.

References

Allison, D. B., Basile, V. C., & MacDonald, R. B. (1991). Brief report: Comparative effects of antecedent exercise and lorazepam on the aggressive behavior of an autistic male. *Journal of Autism and Developmental Disorders, 21*, 89-94.

Aman, M. G., Singh, N. N., Stewart, A. W., & Field, C. J. (1985). The aberrant behavior checklist: A behavior rating scale for the assessment of treatment effects. *American Journal on Mental Deficiency, 89*, 485-491.

Baumeister, A. A., & MacLean, W. E. (1984). Deceleration of self-injurious and stereotypic responding by exercise. *Applied Research in Mental Retardation, 5*, 385-393.

Berkson, G., & Mason, W. A. (1963). Stereotyped movements of mental defectives. III. Situational effects. *American Journal of Mental Deficiency, 68*, 409-412.

Bowman, L. G., Fisher, W. W., Thompson, R. H., & Piazza, C. C. (1997). On the relation of mands and the function of destructive behavior. *Journal of Applied Behavior Analysis, 30*, 251-265.

Carr, E. G. (1977). The motivation of self-injurious behavior: A review of some hypotheses. *Psychological Bulletin, 84*, 800-816.

Carr, E. G., Newsom, C. D., & Binkoff, J. A. (1980). Escape as a factor in the aggressive behavior of two retarded children. *Journal of Applied Behavior Analysis, 13*, 101-117.

Catania, A. C. (1998). *Learning* (4th ed.). Upper Saddle River, NJ: Prentice-Hall.

Catania, A. C., Mathews, B. A., & Shimoff, E. H. (1982). Instructed versus shaped human behavior: Interactions with nonverbal responding. *Journal of the Experimental Analysis of Behavior, 38*, 233-248.

Chapman, S., Fisher, W., Piazza, C. C., & Kurtz, P. F. (1993). Functional assessment and treatment of life-threatening drug ingestion in a dually diagnosed youth. *Journal of Applied Behavior Analysis, 26*, 255-256.

Charlop, M. H., Kurtz, P. F., & Casey, F. G. (1990). Using aberrant behaviors as reinforcers for autistic children. *Journal of Applied Behavior Analysis, 23*, 163-181.

Cooper, L. J., Wacker, D. P., Sasso, G. M., Reimers, T. M., & Donn, L. K. (1990). Using parents as therapists to evaluate appropriate behavior of their children: Application to a tertiary diagnostic clinic. *Journal of Applied Behavior Analysis, 23*, 285-296.

Derby, K. M., Fisher, W. W., & Piazza, C. C. (1996). The effects of contingent and noncontingent attention on self-injury and self-restraint. *Journal of Applied Behavior Analysis, 29*, 101-110.

Derby, K. M., Hagopian, L. P., Fisher, W. W., Augustin, M., Fahs, A., Thompson, R. H., & Owen-DeSchryver, J. (1998). Analyzing multiple topographies of aberrant behavior using functional analysis procedures: A summary of 50 clients. Manuscript in preparation.

Derby, K. M., Wacker, D. P., Sasso, G. M., Steege, M., Northup, J., Cigrand, K., & Asmus, J. (1992). Brief functional assessment techniques to evaluate aberrant behavior in an outpatient setting: A summary of 79 cases. *Journal of Applied Behavior Analysis, 25,* 713-722.

Dunlap, G., Kern-Dunlap, L., Clarke, S., & Robbins, F. R. (1991). Functional assessment, curricular revision, and severe behavior problems. *Journal of Applied Behavior Analysis, 24,* 387-397.

Eisenberger, R., Karpman, M., & Trattner, T. (1967). What is the necessary and sufficient condition for reinforcement in the contingency situation? *Journal of Experimental Psychology, 74,* 342-350.

Fisher, W. W., Adelinis, J. D., Thompson, R. H., Worsdell, A. S., & Zarcone, J. R. (1998). Functional analysis and treatment of destructive behavior maintained by termination of "Don't" (and symmetrical "Do") requests. *Journal of Applied Behavior Analysis, 31,* 339-356.

Fisher, W. W., Lindauer, S. E., Alterson, C. J., & Thompson, R. H. (in press). Assessment and treatment of property destruction automatically maintained by access to preferred stereotypies. *Journal of Applied Behavior Analysis.*

Fisher, W., Piazza, C., Cataldo, M., Harrell, R., Jefferson, G., & Conner, R. (1993). Functional communication training with and without extinction and punishment. *Journal of Applied Behavior Analysis, 26,* 23-36.

Griffin, J. C., Williams, D. E., Stark, M. T., Altmeyer, B. K., & Mason M. (1986). Self-injurious behavior: A state-wide prevalence survey of the extent and circumstances. *Applied Research in Mental Retardation, 7,* 105-116.

Hagopian, L. P., Fisher, W. W., & Legacy, S. M. (1994). Schedule effects of noncontingent reinforcement on attention-maintained destructive behavior in identical quadruplets. *Journal of Applied Behavior Analysis, 27,* 317-325.

Horner, R. H., Day, H. M., & Day, J. R. (1997). Using neutralizing routines to reduce problem behaviors. *Journal of Applied Behavior Analysis, 30,* 601-614.

Horner, R. H., Day, H. M., Sprague, J. R., O'Brien, M., & Heathfield, L. T. (1991). Interspersed requests: A nonaversive procedure for reducing aggression and self-injury during instruction. *Journal of Applied Behavior Analysis, 24,* 265-278.

Iwata, B. A., Dorsey, M. F., Slifer, K. J., Bauman, K. E., & Richman, G. S. (1994). Toward a functional analysis of self-injury. *Journal of Applied Behavior Analysis, 27,* 197-209. (Reprinted from *Analysis and Intervention in Developmental Disabilities, 2,* 3-20, 1982.)

Iwata, B. A., Pace, G. M., Cowdery, G. E., & Miltenberger, R. G. (1994). What makes extinction work: An analysis of procedural form and function. *Journal of Applied Behavior Analysis, 27,* 131-144.

Iwata, B. A., Pace, G. M., Dorsey, M. F., Zarcone, J. R., Vollmer, T. R., Smith, R. G., Rodgers, T. A., Lerman, D. C., Shore, B. A., Mazaleski, J. L., Goh, H., Cowdery, G. E., Kalsher, M. J., McCosh, K. C., & Willis, K. D. (1994). The functions of self-injurious behavior: An experimental-epidemiological analysis. *Journal of Applied Behavior Analysis, 27,* 215- 240.

Kennedy, C. H., & Meyer, K. A. (1996). Sleep deprivation, allergy symptoms, and negatively reinforced problem behavior. *Journal of Applied Behavior Analysis, 29,* 133-135.

Kennedy, C. H., & Souza, G. (1995). Functional analysis and treatment of eye-poking. *Journal of Applied Behavior Analysis, 28,* 27-37.

Konarski, E. A. (1987). Effects of response deprivation on the instrumental performance of mentally retarded persons. *American Journal of Mental Deficiency, 91,* 537-542.

Konarski, E. A., Johnson, M. R., Crowell, C. R., & Whitman, T. I. (1980). Response deprivation and reinforcement in applied settings: A preliminary analysis. *Journal of Applied Behavior Analysis, 13,* 595-609.

Lalli, J. S., Mace, F. C., Wohn, T., & Livezey, K. (1995). Identification and modification of a response-class hierarchy. *Journal of Applied Behavior Analysis, 28,* 551-559.

Laties, V. G., Weiss, B., & Weiss, A. B. (1969). Further observations on overt "mediating" behavior and the discrimination of time. *Journal of the Experimental Analysis of Behavior, 12,* 43-57.

Lovaas, O. I., & Simmons, J. Q. (1969). Manipulation of self-destruction in three retarded children. *Journal of Applied Behavioral Analysis, 2,* 143-157.

Mace, F. C., & Belfiore, P. (1990). Behavioral momentum in the treatment of escape-motivated stereotypy. *Journal of Applied Behavioral Analysis, 23,* 507-514.

Maurice, P., & Trudel, G. (1982). Self-injurious behavior: Prevalence and relationships to environmental events. In J. H. Hollis & C. E. Meyers (Eds.), *Life-threatening behavior: Analysis and intervention* (pp. 81-103). Washington, DC: American Association on Mental Deficiency.

Michael, J. (1993). Establishing operations. *The Behavior Analyst, 16,* 191-206.

Neef, N. A., Shafer, M. S., Egel, A. L., Cataldo, M. F., & Parrish, J. M. (1983). The class specific effects of compliance training with "do" and "don't" requests: Analogue analysis and classroom application. *Journal of Applied Behavior Analysis, 16,* 81-99.

O'Reilly, M. F. (1995). Functional analysis and treatment of escape-maintained aggression correlated with sleep deprivation. *Journal of Applied Behavior Analysis, 28,* 225-226.

Pace, G. M., Iwata, B. A., Cowdery, G. E., Andree, P. J., & McIntyre, T. (1993). Stimulus (instructional) fading during extinction of self-injurious escape behavior. *Journal of Applied Behavior Analysis, 26,* 205-212.

Polson, D. A. D., & Parsons, J. A. (1994). Precurrent contingencies: Behavior reinforced by altering reinforcement probability for other behavior. *Journal of the Experimental Analysis of Behavior, 61,* 427-439.

Powell, S. B., Bodfish, J. W., Parker, D., Crawford, T. W., & Lewis, M. H. (1996). Self-restraint and self-injury: Occurrence and motivational significance. *American Journal on Mental Retardation, 101,* 41-48.

Premack, D. (1965). Reinforcement theory. In D. Levine (Ed.), *Nebraska symposium on motivation* (Vol. 13, pp. 123-180). Lincoln: University of Nebraska Press.

Premack, D. (1971). Catching up with common sense or two sides of a generalization: Reinforcement and punishment. In R. Glaser (Ed.), *The nature of reinforcement.* (pp. 121-150). New York: Academic Press.

Sheffield, F.D., Roby, T.B., & Campbell, B.A. (1954). Drive reduction versus consummatory behavior as determinants of reinforcement. *Journal of Comparative
and Physiological Psychology, 47*, 349-354.

Sigafoos, J., Elkins, J., Kerr, M., & Attwood, T. (1994). A survey of aggressive
behaviour among a population of persons with intellectual disability in
Queensland. *Journal of Intellectual Disability Research, 38*, 369-381.

Skinner, B. F. (1953). *Science and Human Behavior.* New York: MacMillan.

Skinner, B. F. (1957). *Verbal behavior.* New York: Appleton-Century-Crofts.

Smith, R. G., & Iwata, B. A. (1997). Antecedent influences on behavior disorders.
Journal of Applied Behavior Analysis, 30, 343-375.

Smith, R. G., Iwata, B. A., Vollmer, T. R., & Pace, G. M. (1992). On the relationship
between self-injurious behavior and self-restraint. *Journal of Applied Behavior
Analysis, 25*, 433-445.

Smith, R. G., Lerman, D. C., & Iwata, B. A. (1996). Self-restraint as positive reinforcement for self-injurious behavior. *Journal of Applied Behavior Analysis, 29*, 99-102.

Sugai, G., & White, W. J. (1986). Effects of using object self-stimulation as a
reinforcer on the prevocational work rates of an autistic child. *Journal of Autism
and Developmental Disorders, 16*, 459-471.

Thompson, R. H., Fisher, W. W., Piazza, C. C., & Kuhn, D. E. (in press). The
evaluation and treatment of aggression maintained by attention and automatic
reinforcement. *Journal of Applied Behavior Analysis.*

Timberlake, W., & Allison, J. (1974). Response deprivation: An empirical approach
to instrumental performance. *Psychological Review, 81*, 146-164.

Touchette, P. E., MacDonald, R. F., & Langer, S. N. (1985). A scatter plot for
identifying stimulus control of problem behavior. *Journal of Applied Behavior
Analysis, 18*, 343-351.

Vaughn, M. E., & Michael, J. L. (1982). Automatic reinforcement: An important but
ignored concept. *Behaviorism, 10*, 217-228.

Vollmer, T.R. (1994). The concept of automatic reinforcement: Implications for
behavioral research in developmental disabilities. *Research in Developmental
Disabilities, 15*, 187-207.

Vollmer, T. R., Iwata, B. A., Zarcone, J. R., Smith, R. G., & Mazaleski, J. L. (1993).
The role of attention in the treatment of attention-maintained self-injurious
behavior: Noncontingent reinforcement and differential reinforcement of other
behavior. *Journal of Applied Behavior Analysis, 26*, 9-21.

Vollmer, T. R., Marcus, B. A., & Ringdahl, J. E. (1995). Noncontingent escape as
treatment for self-injurious behavior maintained by negative reinforcement.
Journal of Applied Behavior Analysis, 28, 15-26.

Vollmer, T. R., Ringdahl, J. E., Roane, H. S., & Marcus, B. A. (1997). Negative side
effects of noncontingent reinforcement. *Journal of Applied Behavior Analysis, 30*,
161-164.

Wacker, D. P., Harding, J., Cooper, L. J., Derby, K. M., Peck, S., Asmus, J., Berg, W. K., & Brown, K. A. (1996). The effects of meal schedule and quantity on problematic behavior. *Journal of Applied Behavior Analysis, 29,* 79-87.

This manuscript was supported in part by Grant MCJ249149-02 from the Maternal and Child Health Service of the U. S. Department of Health and Human Services.

Discussion of Fisher, Piazza,
Alterson, and Kuhn

Relations Among Aberrant Behaviors Exhibited by Individuals with Autism and Developmental Disabilities

David A. Wilder
University of Nevada, Reno

Fisher, Piazza, Alterson, and Kuhn discussed the ways in which two temporally proximate aberrant behaviors may be related. My discussion of their presentation will focus on three issues. The first issue is the importance of Fisher et al.'s work given the prevalence of temporally proximate aberrant behaviors. The second issue involves the extent to which this work draws upon basic behavior-analytic research. Finally, issues relating to the social validation of behavior-analytic procedures will be discussed.

The Prevalence of Temporally Proximate Aberrant Behavior

It is likely that many of those who have worked with individuals with autism and other developmental disabilities have observed the co-occurrence of two topographically distinct aberrant behaviors. For example, an individual might engage in a form of self-injury (SIB) concurrent with aggression or stereotypy. The scientific literature supports the frequency with which this observation is made. (In the context of the literature on SIB and self-restraint, which is one of the areas in which much applied research on response-response relations has been conducted, it has been shown that up to half of all individuals who exhibit SIB also exhibit self-restraint (e.g., Smith, Iwata, Vollmer, & Pace, 1992). Other research indicates that most individuals with developmental disabilities who display one aberrant behavior display at least one more (e.g., Maurice & Trudel, 1982; Powell, Bodfish, Parker, Crawford, & Lewis, 1986; Sigafoos, Elkins, Kerr, & Attwood, 1994).

Fisher et al. discuss a phenomenon that is relatively common in individuals with autism and other developmental disabilities. Analyzing the relationship between co-occurring aberrant behavior is important because it may lead to improved assessment and treatment efforts for this common phenomenon. An example of these advancements was reported by Smith, Lerman, & Iwata (1996) who developed a method of assessing the extent to which one aberrant behavior functions as reinforcement for another.

Basic Research on Interresponse Relations

One of the prevailing themes of this conference was the emphasis on the relation between basic and applied behavior-analytic research. The research reported by Fisher et al. on temporally proximate aberrant behaviors constitutes a clear exception to the common notion that basic and applied research are not easily integrated. A number of explanations of the relationship between co-occurring aberrant behavior draw directly from the basic research literature. For example, Fisher et al. report that the nature of aberrant response-response relations may involve one aberrant behavior functioning as reinforcement for another aberrant response, as in a case where access to self-restraint functions as reinforcement for SIB. This hypothesis draws upon two theories from the basic literature: the Premack principle, and response deprivation theory. Further, Fisher et al.'s hypothesis on the termination of one aberrant behavior functioning as negative reinforcement for another, as in the case where termination of SIB functions as negative reinforcement for self-restraint, is influenced by the basic work of Terrace (1974). The integration of basic and applied research, as exemplified by Fisher et al., will ensure that our field remains conceptually sound and technically accurate.

The Social Validity of Behavioral Interventions for Aberrant Behavior

Fisher et al. described a number of effective interventions for aberrant interresponse relations. The interventions were conducted in the context of tightly controlled clinical settings. Studies such as these are a testimonial to what can be accomplished with behavioral technology given adequate resources. However, the social validity of some of the procedures conducted under such ideal conditions may be threatened. Threats to the social validity of these interventions center around the lack of resources encountered in typical clinics, schools, and homes. Time, money, and staffing ratios often make the interventions employed in well-controlled settings qualitatively and quantitatively different from those employed in naturalistic settings. It may be that interventions conducted under ideal conditions should also be evaluated in settings that are more naturalistic in order to establish their generality. This is not to say that the procedures developed in well-controlled settings are ineffective, for they have been demonstrated to be effective in the context in which they are conducted. However, in addition to the discovery and evaluation of procedures in tightly controlled settings, applied researchers need to extend the growing intervention research into areas that are less controlled and more closely resemble naturalistic environments.

In conclusion, Fisher et al.'s presentation described a novel program of research involving a common problem among individuals with autism and other developmental disabilities. This research draws on basic theories and findings in behavior analysis to manager the occurrence of aberrant response-response relations. Advances in functional assessment and intervention technology will continue to facili-

tate advances in treatmentsfor co-occurring aberrant behavior. This is an exciting
new area, and it will surely impact our current understanding of aberrant response-
environment relations.

References

Maurice, P., & Trudel, G. (1982). Self-injurious behavior: Prevalence and relationships to environmental events. In J. H. Hollis & C. E. Meyers (Eds.), *Life-
threatening behavior: Analysis and intervention* (pp. 81-103). Washington, DC:
American Association on Mental Deficiency.

Powell, S. B., Bodfish, J. W., Parker, D., Crawford, T. W., & Lewis, M. H. (1996). Self-
restraint and self-injury: Occurrence and motivational significance. *American
Journal on Mental Retardation, 101*, 41-48.

Sigafoos, J., Elkins, J., Kerr, M., & Attwood, T. (1994). A survey of aggressive behavior
among a population of persons with intellectual disability in Queensland.
Journal of Intellectual Disability Research, 28, 369-381.

Smith, R. G., Iwata, B. A., Vollmer, T. R., & Pace, G. M. (1992). On the relationship
between self-injurious behavior and self-restraint. *Journal of Applied Behavior
Analysis, 25*, 433-445.

Smith, R. G., Lerman, D. C., & Iwata, B. A. (1992). Self-restraint as positive reinforcement for self-injurious behavior. *Journal of Applied Behavior Analysis, 29*, 99-102.

Terrace, H. S. (1974). On the nature of nonresponding in discrimination learning
with and without errors. *Journal of the Experimental Analysis of Behavior, 22*, 151-
159.

Chapter 7

The Need for Both Discrete Trial and Natural Environment Language Training for Children With Autism

Mark L. Sundberg and James W. Partington
Behavior Analysts, Inc.

Abstract

Skinner's (1957) analysis of verbal behavior is used to compare discrete trial training (DTT) and natural environment training (NET). These two procedures are frequently cited in the literature on teaching language to children with autism and other developmental disabilities. The results of the analysis show that the two approaches typically focus on different types of verbal behavior. Both teach receptive and expressive language, but NET is primarily based on mand training by incorporating the child's current establishing operations and the delivery of specific reinforcement, while DTT is primarily based on tact and receptive training by using nonverbal and verbal stimuli and nonspecific reinforcement. Intraverbal behavior typically is not a major focus of either approach, but NET seems more conducive to certain types of intraverbal training. A more effective approach to teaching language to children with autism might consist of a combination of DTT and NET procedures, using Skinner's analysis of verbal behavior as a conceptual framework for the intervention, rather than the traditional cognitive framework of language that underlies most treatment programs. Suggestions are made for ways to use Skinner's analysis of verbal behavior, and both DTT and NET, to teach language to children with autism.

Introduction

Children with autism have historically provided unique challenges to the professionals who work with them. Perhaps the most complex task faced by these professionals is the development and implementation of effective language intervention programs. Language is complex, and for many nonverbal children with autism it often requires a substantial amount of skill and effort on the part of parents and teachers to develop a successful communication repertoire. Many specific language skills must be directly taught to these children, and careful programming provided, in order for generalization and spontaneity to occur. In addition, these children eventually need to be able to acquire new types of language skills without highly trained staff or a carefully programmed individualized educational environment. A substantial amount of literature on autism suggests that a behavioral approach can best provide these necessary elements for successful language instruction (Maurice, Green, & Luce, 1996).

However, in the behavioral literature there are several quite different approaches to language instruction for children with autism. Two common approaches have been identified as discrete trial training (e.g., Lovaas, 1981; Lovaas, Koegel, Simmons, & Long, 1983; Smith, 1993), and the natural language paradigm (e.g., Koegel, O'Dell & Koegel, 1987; Laski, Charlop, & Schreibman, 1988). There are several variations of these two different approaches to language training (e.g., Guess, Sailor,

Table 1. Comparison of Discrete Trial Training and Natural Environment Training*

Discrete Trial (Analog)	Natural Environment (NLP)
Stimulus items	
a. Chosen by clinician	a. Chosen by child
b. Repeated until criterion is met	b. Varied every few trials
c. Phonologically easy to produce irrespective of whether they were functional in the natural environment	
Interaction	
a. Clinician holds up stimulus item; stimulus item not functional within interaction	a. Clinician and child play with stimulus item (i.e., stimulus item functional within interaction)
Response	
a. Correct response or successive approximations reinforced	a. Looser shaping contingency so that attempts to respond verbally (except self-stimulation) are also reinforced
Consequences	
a. Edible reinforcers paired with social reinforcers	a. Natural reinforcers (e.g., opportunity to play with the item) paired with social reinforcers

*Adapted from Koegel, Koegel, and Surratt (1992).

& Baer, 1976; Halle, 1987; Hart & Risley, 1975; Kent, 1974; Hart & Rogers-Warren, 1978). Koegel, Koegel, and Surratt (1992) provided a summary of the basic elements of these two approaches (Table 1), and they will be briefly reviewed here.

The main aspect of discrete trial training (DTT), also called analog training by Koegel, et al., (1992) is that language intervention is conducted in a highly specified and structured manner. The instructor chooses and presents a specific stimulus related to a target skill, and when the student responds correctly (perhaps with prompting) the response is reinforced with strong reinforcers such as food. Incorrect responses typically result in the use of a correction procedure, and training on a specific skill is often repeated until a mastery criterion is met. Language skills are divided into a number of independent tasks (or drills), and mass trial training typically occurs in a designated situation (e.g., at a table). In addition, the instructor often presents a command to respond to a specific task in a slightly louder voice, with the clear indication to the child that he is expected to respond. Some approaches to discrete trial training (DTT) recommend punishing non-responding and incorrect responses with verbal reprimands usually in the form of a loud "No!" Discrete trial training can be very effective (e.g., Smith, 1993), especially when compared to the indirect type of language intervention (e.g., large group and activity-based instruction) common to many special education classrooms.

The essential features of natural environment training (NET, also called the Natural Language Paradigm (NLP) by Koegel, et al., (1987) involve focusing on the child's immediate interests and activities as a guide for language instruction. NET is looser and conducted in the child's typical daily environment (e.g., his home, a playground, the community), rather than in a formal teaching arrangement. Stimulus and response variation is stressed, and the consequences for correct verbal responses are specific to the child's interest or activities, rather than consequences that are irrelevant to the response (e.g., giving a child the ball for identifying a ball rather than giving him an M&M). There are a number of language training approaches and techniques that have been based on this general orientation (e.g., incidental teaching, milieu teaching), and these approaches, along with NLP, have been successful in teaching a variety of language delayed children more advanced language skills (e.g., Halle, 1987; Hart & Risley, 1975; Koegel, O'Dell, & Koegel, 1987; Hart & Rogers-Warren, 1978; Warren & Kaiser, 1986).

Both DTT and NET have been shown to be effective. However, these quite different approaches to language instruction have generated a substantial amount of discussion and disagreement among professionals as to which method is the most effective. In a recent series of research, DTT (identified by the authors as analog training) was contrasted with NET (identified by the authors as the natural language paradigm) in an attempt to determine which behavioral approach to language instruction produced better results (Elliot, Hall, & Soper, 1991; Koegel, Koegel, & Surratt, 1992). The findings of these studies were somewhat mixed with Elliot, et al. (1991), who made their assessments under conditions favoring analog training to assure against bias, reporting no statistical difference between the two methods.

However, these authors concluded that "Because natural language teaching has many strengths, few drawbacks, and produces equal generalization and retention under disadvantageous conditions, it is strongly supported as preferable for people with autism and mental retardation" (p. 444). Koegel, et al. (1992), using a different methodology, found that "teaching language to autistic children in a natural teaching context typically produced more correct target behavior than an analog approach. The results also added to the literature by showing that the children exhibited considerably less disruptive behavior during the natural language conditions" (p.151).

Given these results, it would seem that a practitioner should conduct natural language training rather than discrete trial training with children with autism. However, the issue as to which approach is the most effective may not be that simple. First, since there is such a wide variation among children with autism, no single approach would probably work for all children. Second, a fundamental problem with the different behavioral approaches to language training presented in the literature (such as the two described above) is that they are not based on a behavioral analysis of language. Rather, while they employ behavioral techniques (e.g., prompting, reinforcement) to teach language skills, they (often unknowingly) are guided by a traditional cognitive or biological analysis of language (e.g., Brown, 1973; Chomsky, 1957; Piaget, 1926; Pinker, 1994). Unfortunately, these traditional analyses of language tend to neglect important environmental variables, and often blend useful distinctions that might be essential to guiding language intervention programs for children with autism. The use of the traditional distinctions between expressive and receptive language common to most of the above-cited research is a hallmark of these traditional analyses of language.

The purpose of the current paper is to further examine DTT and NET, but with the help of Skinner's (1957) functional analysis of verbal behavior. Skinner's analysis of verbal behavior has been used as a conceptual tool to help analyze a variety of topics in the analysis of language, such as the acquisition of language by children (e.g., Bijou & Baer, 1965), the acquisition of language by apes (e.g., Savage-Rumbaugh, 1984; Sundberg, 1996), language assessment (Partington & Sundberg, 1998; Spradlin, 1963; Sundberg, 1983), the use of Facilitated Communication (e.g., Hall, 1993; Sundberg, 1993), stimulus equivalence (e.g., Hall & Chase, 1991), and schizophrenic hallucinations (e.g., Burns, Heiby, & Tharp, 1983; Layng & Andronis, 1984). There are many theoretical analyses of language available to the professional, but Skinner's analysis of language, and its focus on environmental variables, can be a valuable guide for the assessment and development of a language intervention program.

The essential feature of Skinner's analysis of verbal behavior is that language is learned behavior under the control of a variety of different environmental variables. Skinner identifies and functionally classifies these different types of environmental variables, and has suggested a number of different verbal operants. Table 2 contains Skinner's technical definitions of each type of verbal behavior (for more detail see Michael, 1982; Sundberg & Partington, 1998; or Winokur, 1976). In general, Skinner goes beyond the traditional classification of receptive and expressive language by distinguishing between receptive language, and 5 functionally independent types of expressive language (echoic/motor imitation/copying-a-text, mand, tact, intraverbal, textual/transcriptive). There are also many subtypes, extensions, and combinations of these basic "elementary verbal operants," as Skinner calls them. The distinction between the mand, tact, and intraverbal is quite complex, and thus frequently not recognized by professionals. However, this distinction often reveals important information regarding the pragmatic aspects of expres-

Table 2. Technical Definitions of Skinner's (1957)
Elementary Verbal Operants

CONTROLLING VARIABLES	RESPONSE	CONSEQUENCE
Verbal stimulus with point-to-point correspondence and formal similarity	Echoic Imitation Copying-a-text	Nonspecific reinforcement
Nonverbal stimulus	Tact	Nonspecific reinforcement
Establishing operations	Mand	Specific reinforcement
Verbal stimulus without point-to point correspondence or formal similarity	Intraverbal	Nonspecific reinforcement
Verbal stimulus with point-to-point correspondence, but without formal similarity	Textual Transcriptive	Nonspecific reinforcement
Verbal stimulus	Nonverbal Response (Receptive language)	Nonspecific reinforcement

Table 3. A Comparison of Discrete Trial Training and Natural Environment Training Using Skinner's Elementary Verbal Operants

	Discrete Trial Training	Natural Environment Training
Mand	Not specifically trained, EO not used, specific reinforcement not used, focus on establishing verbal and nonverbal stimulus control	Focus on establishing operations and use of specific reinforcement Multiply controlled if verbal or nonverbal stimuli present
Receptive	Specifically trained, focus on verbal and nonverbal stimulus control	Specifically trained, but multiply controlled if EO, and contextual stimuli present
Tact	Specifically trained, focus on nonverbal stimulus control	Specifically trained, but multiply controlled if EO and specific reinforcement present
Echoic	Specifically trained, focus on vocal verbal stimulus control	Specifically trained, but multiply controlled if EO, nonverbal stimuli, and specific reinforcement present
Imitation	Specifically trained, focus on visual motor stimulus control	Specifically trained, but multiply controlled if EO, nonverbal stimuli, and specific reinforcement present
Intraverbal	Not specifically trained, multiply controlled if EO, object, and specific reinforcement present	Specifically trained, but multiply controlled if EO, nonverbal stimuli, and specific reinforcement present

sive communication, especially for the analysis of defective or delayed language skills.

By using Skinner's elementary verbal operants as a tool to classify the types of language behavior focused on in training, the distinction between DTT and NET can be more closely examined. Table 3 contains a comparison of the two approaches across the different elementary verbal operants.

Mand

Perhaps the most significant difference between DTT and NET is that NET primarily involves the basic elements of mand training (i.e., the use of establishing operations and specific reinforcement), while DTT primarily involves the basic elements of receptive, tact, echoic, and imitation training (i.e., verbal and nonverbal stimulus control, and nonspecific reinforcement). There is an extensive body of research on the many differences between mand training and training on the other types of verbal behavior (for reviews see Oah & Dickenson, 1987; Shafer, 1994; Brady, Saunders, & Spradlin, 1994). Perhaps the most important distinction between these types of verbal behavior is the role of the establishing operation (EO) as an independent variable controlling the mand (Michael, 1988, 1993). Previous research has shown that use of the EOs and specific reinforcement can facilitate language acquisition (e.g., Braam & Sundberg, 1991; Carroll & Hesse, 1987; Hall & Sundberg, 1987; Stafford, Sundberg, & Braam, 1987). From a practical point of view, language training can be a lot more successful and fun for children if their ongoing establishing operations guide language intervention, especially for manding. However, as will be discussed shortly, children must also learn verbal behaviors not solely related to their current EOs.

Receptive, Tact, Echoic, and Imitation

Much of typically developing children's language is controlled by what they see and hear in their daily environment. Receptive, tact, echoic, and imitation are types of verbal behavior that are evoked by these verbal and nonverbal stimuli in that environment. DTT may be more suited for teaching these types of verbal behavior because of the high rate of trials often required, and the absence of the EO as a source of control in training. In fact, it may be possible that training in the absence of the EO helps the child learn how to work and attend for extended periods of time, which is required for success in a typical classroom. However, it is often the case that strong forms of reinforcement, or even mild aversive control, are needed to make this type of instruction successful because many of the tasks are irrelevant to the child's current EOs, and are out of context.

Receptive, tact, echoic, and imitation training can also be conducted with NET, but including EOs and specific reinforcement as variables that may facilitate the acquisition of these skills (e.g., Carroll & Hesse, 1987). However, it may be difficult to conduct a high rate of training trials, and a special effort must be made to ensure that the responses ultimately are not multiply controlled by EOs and specific reinforcement. For example, a child might be successful at receptively identifying a Winnie the Pooh video tape in a natural context, but his success may be multiply controlled by not only the video and the verbal instruction, but also by the establishing operations related to the video, the presence of other stimuli associated with the video (e.g., a VCR, TV), and getting to watch the video. It should be pointed out that multiple control is not necessarily undesireable; in fact, these additional variables may facilitate the initial acquisition of some types of language. However, the problem with multiple control is that EOs, specific reinforcement, and other forms of verbal and nonverbal stimulus control, may not be present outside of the original NET conditions, thus possibly reducing the probability of generalizing these types of verbal responses to less interesting, but still important, environmental conditions.

Intraverbal

Intraverbal behavior is not a major focus in the early phases of either approach. However, training on this verbal skill is essential for the development of conversations, social interaction, and certain types of academic behavior. NET seems more conducive to intraverbal training, and procedures are often included to increase intraverbal responding (e.g., "expansion" in incidental teaching). However, when intraverbal behavior is taught, both approaches may unintentionally develop multiply controlled responding if training does not include conditions where the EO, specific reinforcement, and nonverbal stimuli are eliminated as independent variables (i.e., the child ultimately needs to acquire pure intraverbal behavior).

A comparison between DTT and NET shows that these two approaches focus on different types of verbal behavior. Both teach receptive and expressive language, but Skinner's analysis of verbal behavior shows that NET primarily involves mand training by incorporating the child's current establishing operations and the delivery of specific reinforcement. DTT primarily involves tact, receptive, echoic, and imitation training by using nonverbal and verbal stimuli and nonspecific reinforcement. However, intraverbal behavior typically is not a major focus of either approach. Since elements of each type of training can benefit children with autism, a more effective approach might consist of a combination of DTT and NET, with intervention programs guided by Skinner's analysis of verbal behavior as a conceptual framework (Sundberg & Partington, 1998). The practical advantages and disadvantages of DTT and NET will now be examined in order to identify further the strengths and weaknesses of each approach. Some of these advantages and disadvantages are presented in Tables 4-7. Other comparisons of DTT and NET are available in the literature, and the reader is referred to these for additional information (e.g., Elliot, Hall, & Soper, 1991; Spradlin & Siegel, 1982).

Advantages of DTT. Perhaps the main advantage of DTT is that a high rate of training trials on specific verbal operants can be conducted. With this clear focus and emphasis on specific language skills, the training program is easier to script, and staff who have only minimal training can conduct the procedures. The training stimuli (e.g., specific target items to label) can be clearly identified and collected prior to training sessions, the targeted responses are measurable and easy to take data on, and the consequences are easy to deliver (e.g., food). In addition, this type of training is more conducive to a classroom structure where it is often impossible to follow each child's EO as it occurs. Thus, it is possible that this arrangement is an effective way to teach those types of verbal behaviors that are not related to the EO and specific reinforcement, or skills that may need an extensive number of training trials to acquire.

Disadvantages of DTT. There are a number of disadvantages of DTT that should be considered (Table 5). While DTT may facilitate a child's acquisition of

---

Table 4. The Advantages of Discrete Trial Training

---

1. Allows for a high number of training trials
2. Easy for many different staff members to implement (a scripted curriculum is used)
3. May be a good way to develop tact, receptive, echoic, and imitative behaviors
4. Easier to run in a classroom setting
5. Instructional stimuli and detailed curriculum provided for staff
6. Target responses are known and easily identified
7. Contrived consequence is easy to deliver
8. Data collection is relatively straight forward
9. Progressive steps in the curriculum clearly identified (e.g., nouns, verbs, pronouns)
10. Progress (or the lack of progress) is very observable
11. May help to establish stimulus control of "learner repertoires" (e.g., child learns to attend, learns that if he does respond he gets reinforced, learns how to make discriminations, learns to sit and work, acquires an increased tolerance of demands)

---

specific verbal responses, the formal structure of the language interaction is often substantially different from that found in the natural environment. The natural environment does not contain strong prompts to respond, (including an implicit requirement that one must respond), nor does it always contain the immediate delivery of powerful reinforcers. Therefore, extensive efforts to establish generalization and thin out reinforcement must be included in the program. In addition, DTT is primarily teacher initiated, and does not make use of the child's on-going EOs, not only neglecting opportunities to teach mands, but also possibly contributing to potential behavior problems. Another disadvantage of DTT is that the drill nature of the training may generate rote responding, and inhibit spontaneous verbal behavior because of the tight stimulus control that is often established. Also, specific skills are typically isolated and taught independently (e.g., tacting, imitation, receptive), however, in typical verbal interactions the different types of verbal behavior (e.g., receptive, mand, tact, intraverbal) are mixed together in a conversation. Also, the interaction between a speaker and listener in the natural environment is very different from the interaction observed in standard DTT (e.g., where the instructor commands each specific response from the child).

Advantages of NET. There are several advantages of conducting language instruction in a child's natural environment (Table 6). Perhaps the most significant variable is the use of the child's current motivation (establishing operations) and the immediate environmental context as guides for the language training process. This

---

Table 5. The Disadvantages of Discrete Trial Training

---

1. Requires special procedures to ensure generalization
2. Prompts to respond (including mild aversive prompts) often not present outside of the training session
3. Child's current EOs not used in training, may even compete with training
4. Mainly teacher initiated activities
5. Mand training is difficult because it requires using EOs and specific reinforcement
6. Intraverbal behavior typically not taught as a separate verbal operant
7. Immediate and powerful reinforcers often not available outside of the training session
8. The drill nature of the training may generate rote responding
9. Non-functional nature of the training may generate escape and avoidance behaviors (possibly increasing the need for the use of aversive control or powerful contrived reinforcers)
10. The interaction between the speaker and listener is very different from that observed by typical speakers and listeners
11. Language and language trainers may become paired with aversive situations
12. Trials that are presented in a scripted manner reduces the trainer's ability to expand on responses or mix the verbal operants, as in typical verbal interactions

---

type of training not only teaches manding, but reduces the need for elaborate generalization procedures, because the training is conducted in the context of natural events in the child's daily environment which are typically the focus of generalization procedures used in DTT (e.g., Koegel & Johnson, 1989; Koegel, et al., 1992). In addition, the child may exhibit fewer negative behaviors because of the focus on his motivation, and the use of consequences directly related to that motivation (Hall & Sundberg, 1987; Stafford, Sundberg, & Braam, 1988; Koegel, Koegel, & Surratt, 1992). NET may also promote more spontaneous verbal behavior because of the focus on EO control rather than trainer SD control.

A skillful trainer can use EOs and specific reinforcement to teach tacts, intraverbals, and other important verbal and nonverbal skills (Sundberg & Partington, 1998). For example, if a child shows interest in playing with a train set it may be quite easy to teach the mand "train," as well as tacts for items related to the train such as track, light, caboose, engine, wheels, etc., and intraverbals such as "It's a choo choo ...." This teaching strategy not only allows the instructor to teach each type of verbal behavior, but the instructor can more easily bring together these different types of verbal behavior as they relate to the current environmental context (e.g., the presence of a train set). This type of interaction typically does not occur in DTT.

Table 6. The Advantages of Natural Environment Training

---

1. Use of the child's interests (EOs) to guide language instruction
2. Best conditions to teach manding
3. Use of the stimuli in the child's natural environment as target SDs
4. Reduced need for elaborate generalization procedures
5. Reduced amount of negative behavior
6. Reduced need for aversive control
7. Easier to teach intraverbal behavior as a separate verbal operant
8. The verbal interaction is much more characteristic of typical verbal interactions
9. More opportunities for trainers to be paired with successful verbal interactions
10. Verbal responses can be mixed together more easily under the environmental conditions that may evoke them later
11. The training conditions are closer to those of kindergarten or other educational environments, and how the child may be taught in the future

---

Disadvantages of NET. There are a number of disadvantages to NET as well (Table 7). Perhaps the main problem is that extra effort must be made to eliminate the EO, specific reinforcement, and other contextual prompts from the language training activities. Attempts to conduct only tact or intraverbal training may be less successful because of the absence of EOs and specific consequences in a language training session. Therefore, conducting language training in the natural environment requires a sophisticated set of skills on the part of the language trainer/parent to move beyond this type of multiply controlled manding. Teaching staff exactly how to conduct this training is much more complicated, because it is hard to predict the child's EOs and behaviors, and there is no scripted curriculum for the teacher to follow. In addition, the amount or training trials and the types of training activities may be limited in the natural environment because the child's interests may be limited, and because of the often cumbersome and time consuming nature of delivering specific reinforcement (e.g., "Take me swimming").

Using primarily the child's EOs to initiate and guide language interactions may be a sharp contrast with the daily contingencies in the child's real world. The child may be required to follow the adult's EOs, and comply with adult's verbal stimuli, while his EOs are ignored or are not understood (as is probably the case with a substantial number of early parent-child relationships). While strong EOs may provide good opportunities to teach more advanced language skills and should be capitalized on, the child must also be able to comply to specific educational routines and instructions delivered by a teacher if the child is to succeed in a typical classroom (Lovaas, 1977). That is, teaching language also involves the establishment of nonverbal (tact) and verbal (receptive, intraverbal, textual) stimulus con-

Table 7. The Disadvantages of Natural Environment Training

1. Training is difficult to conduct in a formal classroom
2. Must be able to capture or contrive on-going EOs
3. Child's EO may be unknown to the trainer
4. Cumbersome to always follow the child's EO
5. Cumbersome to always deliver specific reinforcement
6. May be difficult to eliminate the role of the EO as a source of control
7. Requires better training on the part of staff
8. Curriculum is not scripted so it is more difficult to know what to do
9. Data collection (measures of acquisition) is much more complicated
10. Substantially reduced number of training trials
11. Training may compete with the establishment of other types of stimulus control

trol. In fact, for some children an extensive focus on their EOs (mands) may interfere with the establishment of these other types of antecedent control, especially verbal stimulus control (e.g., compliance, receptive discriminations).

Combining DTT and NET for Daily Language Instruction

Language intervention for children with autism should involve teaching all the different elementary verbal operants, under a variety of environmental contexts, while being assured that each type of verbal behavior can stand on its own, and can be mixed together (Skinner, 1957; Sundberg & Partington, 1998). For example, the success of a child's tact repertoire should not be dependent on the presence of mand variables (i.e., EOs and specific reinforcement), just like the tact should be able to lead to a relevant intraverbal, if the conditions warrant it. DTT and NET are both effective procedures, and each offers specific advantages for teaching certain types of verbal behavior. The exclusive use of only one of these approaches may be less effective than a combination of the two when guided by Skinner's analysis of verbal behavior.

Unfortunately, the terms that have evolved as descriptors for these two approaches are somewhat misleading. Technically, a "discrete trial" is a three-term contingency consisting of a stimulus-response-consequence relationship (e.g., staff hold up a car—child says "car"—staff says "right!"). Recently however, "discrete trial" has come to be used by parents and educators as a descriptor for an entire approach to language instruction, usually that of Lovaas. However, discrete trials are not restricted to the implementation of an entire program (which is often requested by parents), but can be conducted in a variety of environmental situations with substantial variation (e.g., Leaf, 1997).

"Natural language" is also a term that suggests other possible meanings. For example, it may suggest linguistically interacting with the child in a manner similar to how one would interact with a typically developing child in a non-educational environment. However, if the child is nonverbal or is limited in his verbal abilities, the informal and casual language instruction provided by parents of typical children may be markedly inadequate for a child with autism (much of the work on incidental and milieu training, which preceded NLP, was conducted with higher functioning children).

However, for many children an effective way of teaching them the different types of verbal behavior is to use the elements of the child's natural environment (i.e., current EOs, events, activities, materials) to conduct intensive training using a discrete trials format. The term "natural environment" is not much better, but seems at least to put the focus on the child's immediate environment, rather than on developmental processes.

There are two general instructional settings for most children with autism: a special education classroom provided by the local school district, and the child's home environment. Language training on all the elementary verbal operants should be conducted in both of these environments, using both DTT and NET techniques. However, depending on the child and the available staff, it may be easier to conduct more DTT in the child's classroom, and more NET in the child's home and community. In the classroom, higher rates of responding can be obtained by sharply increasing the rate of reinforcement and producing not only faster acquisition, but also better instructional control by the staff. It is also hard to follow each child's EO and deliver specific reinforcement all the time in a classroom setting. In addition, if a child is to succeed independently in the typical educational system, he or she needs to acquire appropriate classroom behaviors.

It is relatively easier to conduct NET in the child's home because the child's EOs can be followed, and specific reinforcement delivered, more easily than in a classroom environment. Also, a wider variety of the stimuli associated with verbal behavior can be accessed for training (e.g., lights, toys, people, sounds, smells). However, at home there is much less of a demand on the child than at school (as is of course the case for typical children); thus, high demand tasks (such as language training for some low verbal children) might be difficult to complete. In addition, DTT may be more difficult at home because reinforcers may be less effective in that are often available noncontingently at home. However, the careful use of EOs to conduct discrete trial training on mands and other types of verbal behavior (with discrete trials), can generate a substantial amount of verbal behavior.

Finally, it is most important to consider the existing skills of the individual child when determining how best to approach his language needs. The balance between DTT and NET may change frequently during the language acquisition process, but training should always include both approaches. Five general phases are suggested, but blends and overlaps of these phases may vary widely with each child (Table 8). During the first phase of language intervention for, say, a nonverbal 3 year old who rarely sits down, a trainer may be more successful following the child's EOs (by capturing and contriving them) and attempting to shape manding (thus, more like NET). Discrete trials are a key part of this training, but they are discrete mand training trials (Sundberg & Partington, 1998). During this phase, NET also allows the instructors to pair themselves with reinforcing activities, rather than with the potential aversive stimuli often associated with formal DTT responding. Mands can be interspersed with other types of trials (e.g., receptive, echoic, imitation) in an effort to begin establishing stimulus control in addition to EO control (Michael, 1982). While a majority of the training may be conducted in the child's natural environment, some DTT training can begin to occur at a table or on the floor.

In Phase 2, the other verbal operants should become more of a focus of training, but mand training should still be conducted at every opportunity. Training should be conducted with both types of general approaches, but during this phase the child should be learning how to work for extended periods of time in a formal language session conducted at a table or desk. In Phase 3, more focus should be placed on the acquisition of academic-like behaviors such as letters and numbers, and more complex language relations such as prepositions and adjectives. Training on these more complex skills (which are often quite unrelated to a child's current EOs) should be conducted at a table or desk, and for extended period of time (e.g., 15-20 minutes between breaks). NET can still be used to teach and help generalize these academic skills and should still be conducted whenever possible.

The objectives of Phase 4 and Phase 5 are to move the child closer to a less restrictive and more typical educational setting. Once the child has acquired a substantial amount of verbal behavior, it is important to teach him how to learn new

Table 8. The Changing Emphasis of DTT and NET as the Child Learns Language

Phase 1. NET > DTT	Focus on early manding, pairing, compliance, stimulus control
Phase 2. NET = DTT	Focus on mand, tact, receptive, imitation, echoic, and intraverbal
Phase 3. DTT > NET	Focus on academic activities and specific skill development
Phase 4. NET > DTT	Focus on learning from group instruction, from peers, and without a highly structured learning environment, training is more like that of typical kindergarten and 1st grade classrooms
Phase 5. DTT > NET	Focus on academic skills and structured learning characteristic of later elementary classrooms

verbal responses from the natural environment (actually this training should be occurring to some degree all along). That is, the child should be able to learn language in the absence of a specific language training structure (e.g., group instruction, activity-based instruction), and from peers. Many of the activities in a typical kindergarten and 1st grade classrooms are of this type, and have the major advantages of typically speaking peers. Phase 5 suggests a shift back to more structured educational activities characteristic of typical late elementary school classrooms.

In conclusion, both DTT and NET can be effective for teaching receptive and expressive language to children with autism. However, a functional analysis of the skills focused on in training shows that these two procedures target different types of expressive language. NET is primarily based on mand training by incorporating the child's current establishing operations and the delivery of specific reinforcement, while DTT is primarily based on tact, receptive, echoic, and imitative training by using nonverbal and verbal stimuli and nonspecific reinforcement. Intraverbal training is not a major focus of either approach, but is an essential type of verbal behavior. A more complete approach to teaching language to children with autism may consist of a combination of DTT and NET procedures, with Skinner's (1957) analysis of verbal behavior as a conceptual framework for the intervention program.

References

Bijou, S. W., & Baer, D. M. (1965). *Child development II: Universal stage of infancy.* Englewood Cliffs, NJ: Prentice-Hall.

Braam, S., & Sundberg, M. L., (1991). The effects of specific versus nonspecific reinforcement on verbal behavior. *The Analysis of Verbal Behavior, 9,* 19-28.

Brady, N. C., Saunders, K. J., & Spradlin, J. E. (1994). A conceptual analysis of request teaching procedures for individuals with severely limited verbal repertoires. *The Analysis of Verbal Behavior, 12,* 43-54.

Brown, R. (1973). *A first language: The early stages.* Cambridge, MA: Harvard University Press.

Burns, C. E. S., Heiby, E. M., & Tharp, R. G. (1983). A verbal behavior analysis of auditory hallucinations. *The Behavior Analyst, 6,* 133-143.

Carroll, R. J., & Hesse, B. E. (1987). The effects of alternating mand and tact training on the acquisition of tacts. *The Analysis of Verbal Behavior, 5,* 55-65.

Charlop-Christy, M. H., & Kelso, S. E. (1996). *How to treat the child with autism.* Claremont CA: Claremont McKenna College Press.

Chomsky, N. (1957). *Syntactic structures.* The Hague: Mouton and Company.

Elliott, R. O. Jr., Hall, K., & Soper, H. V. (1991). Analog language teaching versus natural language teaching: Generalization and retention of language learning for adults with autism and mental retardation. *Journal of Autism and Developmental Disorders, 21,* 433-447.

Guess, D., Sailor, W. S., & Baer, D. M. (1976). *A functional speech and language program for the severely retarded.* Lawrence KS: H & H Enterprises.

Hall, G. A. (1993). Facilitator control as automatic behavior: A verbal behavior analysis. *The Analysis of Verbal Behavior, 11,* 89-97.

Hall, G. A., & Chase, P. N. (1991). The relationship between stimulus equivalence and verbal behavior. *The Analysis of Verbal Behavior, 9,* 107-119.

Hall, G. A., & Sundberg, M. L. (1987). Teaching mands by manipulating conditioned establishing operations. *The Analysis of Verbal Behavior, 5,* 41-53.

Halle, J. (1987). Teaching language in the natural environment: An analysis of spontaneity. *Journal of the Association for Persons with Severe Handicaps, 12,* 28-37.

Hart, B., & Rogers-Warren, A. (1978). A milieu approach to language teaching. In R. Schiefelbusch (Ed.), *Language intervention strategies* (pp. 193-235). Baltimore, MD: University Park Press.

Hart B., & Risley T. R. (1975). Incidental teaching of language in the preschool. *Journal of Applied Behavior Analysis, 8,* 411-420.

Kent, L. (1974). *Language acquisition program for the retarded or multiply impaired.* Champaign, IL: Research Press.

Koegel, R. L., & Johnson, J. (1989). Motivating language use in autistic children. In G. Dawson (Ed.), *Autism: Nature, diagnosis, and treatment* (pp. 310-325). New York: Guilford.

Koegel, R. L., Koegel, L. K., & Surratt, A. (1992). Language intervention and disruptive behavior in preschool children with autism. *Journal of Autism and Developmental Disorders, 22,* 141-153.

Koegel, R. L., O'Dell, M. C., & Koegel, L. K. (1987). A natural language teaching paradigm for nonverbal autistic children. *Journal of Autism and Developmental Disorders, 17,* 187-200.

Laski, K. E., Charlop, M. H., & Schreibman, L. (1988). Training parents to use the natural language paradigm to increase their autistic children's speech. *Journal of Applied Behavior Analysis, 21,* 391-400.

Layng, T. V. J., & Andronis, P. T. (1984). Toward a functional analysis of delusional speech and hallucinatory behavior. *The Behavior Analyst, 7,* 139-156.

Leaf, R. (February, 1997). *Illusions, delusions, and conclusions of discrete trial training.* Symposium conducted at the 15th Annual Conference of the Northern California Association for Behavior Analysis, Oakland, CA.

Lovaas, O. I. (1977). *The autistic child: Language development through behavior modification.* New York: Irvington.

Lovaas, O. I. (1981). *Teaching developmentally disabled children: The ME book.* Baltimore: University Park Press.

Lovaas, O. I., Koegel, R., Simmons, J.Q., & Long, J. (1973). Some generalization and follow-up measures on autistic children in behavior therapy. *Journal of Applied Behavior Analysis, 6,* 131-166.

Maurice, C., Green, G., & Luce, S.C. (1996). *Behavior interventions for young children with autism.* Austin, Texas: Pro Ed.

Michael, J. (1982). Distinguishing between discriminative and motivational functions of stimuli. *Journal of the Experimental Analysis of Behavior, 37,* 149-155.

Michael, J. (1988). Establishing operations and the mand. *The Analysis of Verbal Behavior, 6,* 3-9.

Michael, J. (1993). Establishing operations. *The Behavior Analyst, 16,* 191-206.

Oah, S., & Dickinson, A. M. (1989). A review of empirical studies of verbal behavior. *The Analysis of Verbal Behavior, 7,* 53-68.

Partington, J.W., & Sundberg, M. L. (1998). *The assessment of basic language and learning skills.* Pleasant Hill, CA: Behavior Analysts, Inc.

Piaget, J. (1926). *The language and thought of the child.* (M. Cook translation). London: Routledge and Kegan Paul, Ltd.

Pinker, S. (1994). *The language instinct.* New York: William Morrow & Company

Savage-Rumbaugh, E. S. (1984). Verbal behavior at the procedural level in the Chimpanzee. *Journal of the Experimental Analysis of Behavior, 41,* 223-250.

Shafer, E. (1994). A review of interventions to teach a mand repertoire. *The Analysis of Verbal Behavior, 12,* 53-66.

Skinner, B. F. (1957). *Verbal Behavior.* New York: Appleton-Century-Crofts.

Smith (1993). Autism. In T. R. Giles (Ed.) *Effective Psychotherapies* (pp. 107-133). New York: Plenum.

Spradlin, J. E. (1963). Assessment of speech and language of retarded children: The Parsons language sample. *Journal of Speech and Hearing Disorders Monograph,10,* 8-31.

Spradlin, J., & Siegel, G. (1982). Language training in natural and clinical environments. *Journal of Speech and Hearing Disorders, 47,* 2-6.

Stafford, M. W., Sundberg, M. L., & Braam, S. (1988). A preliminary investigation of the consequences that define the mand and the tact. *The Analysis of Verbal Behavior, 6,* 61-71.

Sundberg, M. L. (1983). Language. In J. L. Matson, & S. E. Breuning (Eds.), *Assessing the mentally retarded* (pp. 285-310). New York: Grune & Stratton.

Sundberg, M. L. (1993). Selecting a response form for nonverbal persons: Facilitated communication, pointing systems, or sign language? *The Analysis of Verbal Behavior, 11,* 99-116.

Sundberg, M. L. (1996). Toward granting linguistic competence to apes: A review of Savage-Rumbaugh, et al. Language comprehension in ape and child. *Journal of the Experimental Analysis of Behavior, 65,* 477-492.

Sundberg, M. L., & Partington, J. W. (1998). *Teaching language to children with autism and other developmental disabilities.* Pleasant Hill, CA: Behavior Analysts, Inc.

Warren, S. F., & Kaiser, A. P. (1986). Incidental language teaching: A critical review. *Journal of Speech and Hearing Disorders, 51,* 291-299.

Winokur, S. (1976). *A primer on verbal behavior.* Englewood Cliffs, NJ: Prentice-Hall.

The authors gratefully acknowledge Cindy Sundberg for her comments on earlier versions of this paper.

Discussion of Sundberg and Partington

How Much Discrete Trial Versus Natural Language Training is Appropriate for Teaching Language to Children with Autism?

Anne R. Cummings

W. L. Williams and Associates

Whereas the experimental analysis of behavior is often considered to have started with B. F. Skinner's work in the mid-thirties, most consider a behavioral treatment of language to have been undertaken much later. However, as Michael (1984) has stated: "While Skinner was working on the basic methods and relations that would be reported in *The Behavior of Organisms* in 1938, he was already convinced that these same principles were necessary and sufficient for understanding human language. He dates the beginning of his systematic work on language as 1934" (p. 2). Before Skinner published *Verbal Behavior* (1957), Joel Greenspoon (1955) developed a method for the experimental investigation of the effect of social reinforcement on human vocal behavior. He had experimenters (as listeners in conversations) verbally reinforce subjects' emissions of plural nouns under conditions of social reinforcement and its absence. The observed control in the relative frequency of plural nouns was taken as evidence that verbal behavior, like other human behavior, was also sensitive to its consequences (operant conditioning). Subsequently, several studies appeared confirming that infants' vocal behavior was affected by its consequences: Brackbill (1958); Haugan and McIntire (1972); Rheingold, Gewirtz and Ross (1959); Routh (1969); Smith, Michael and Sundberg (1995); Todd and Palmer (1968); Weisberg (1963). Over the next twenty years, there were many documented studies examining specific aspects of verbal repertoires such as their grammatical characteristics (Guess, Sailor, Rutherford, & Baer, 1968; Hart & Risley, 1968; Sailor & Taman, 1972); remedial instruction (Baer & Guess, 1971; Keller & Bucher, 1979); non-vocal (sign) repertoires (Faw, Reid, Schepis, Fitzgerald, & Welty, 1981) and relations between verbal and non-verbal behavior (Israel, 1978). Additionally, it became apparent with the initial studies of Baer and Sherman (1964), Metz (1965), and the work of Peterson (1968), that imitation is crucial to acquiring new verbal behavior, and that the role of reinforcement in the development of generalized imitation was pivotal to the understanding of normal language acquisition.

The study of verbal behavior has been prominent in the field of the experimental analysis of behavior for almost as long as the field itself has existed. In Osgood's

(1958) review of Skinner's *Verbal Behavior,* he called it "one of the two or three most significant contributions to this field in our time" (p. 212). Thirty years later, Jack Michael (1988) described Skinner's analysis of language as "a major behavioral breakthrough, with many theoretical and practical implications" (p. 9). Oah and Dickenson (1989) reviewed empirical research that had been directly influenced by Skinner's *Verbal Behavior.* They found that, "despite the importance of this subject matter, there has been relatively little empirical research conducted in this area" (p.1).

For almost as long as dilemmas have been studied in normal language acquisition, dilemmas have been studied in the language acquisition of children with autism. While some see autism primarily as a deficit in social behavior, others view it primarily as a communication disorder. Needless to say, deficits in language behavior comprise perhaps the most serious problem in autistic children. Professionals supporting children with autism are constantly challenged effectively to develop, implement, and train others in language acquisition skills. No one would argue that the failure to use language to communicate constitutes a profound deficit, and one that has serious and pervasive ramifications for other areas of development. Yet a major current challenge for professionals is the programming for generalization and spontaneity in language for children with autism.

As Schreibman (1988) has observed, "studies have indicated that individuals who develop some language and communicative facilities early in life (i.e. by the age of five years) have a much better clinical prognosis than those who do not (Eisenberg & Kanner, 1956; Rutter, 1968). Given this information, it is certainly understandable that a substantial proportion of the experimental work in the treatment of autism has focused on language" (p. 106). As summarized by Green (1996), there have been many studies showing that behavioral intervention can produce large improvements in specific and important areas related to language, such as peer interaction and classroom behavior (Strain, Hoyson and Jamieson, 1985); imitation (Young, Krantz, McClannahan & Poulson, 1994); self-care (Pierce & Schreibman, 1994); various language skills (Lovaas, 1987, Taylor & Harris, 1995); and home-based behavioral intervention (Lovaas 1987, Lovaas & Smith 1988).

The chapter by Sundberg and Partington redirects us back to the basics in the dilemmas of language training. To date, there have been several studies demonstrating improved instructional techniques in language training for children with learning difficulties, such as increasing motivation (Dunlap, 1984); the use of direct reinforcers (Keogel, 1987); frequently varying tasks and stimulus materials (Dunlap, 1984); reinforcing verbal attempts to communicate (Keogel, 1987); and using incidental teaching (Carr, 1983; Hart & Risley, 1980). There have also been studies demonstrating the benefits of a variety of modified incidental teaching procedures such as the natural language teaching paradigm (Keogel, 1987); delay procedures (Halle, Marshall & Spradlin, 1979); interruption of established behavior chains (Goetz, Gee & Sailor, 1985); loose training (Campbell, 1982) and embedded instruction (Neef, 1984). Sundberg and Partington summarize such modified procedures with a term they coin as "natural environment training" (a term that suggests encompassing a variety of the above-described techniques). Additionally, the litera-ture contains studies comparing discrete trial training methods to a variety of natural language procedures (Elliott, Hall & Soper, 1991; McGee, Krantz & McClannahan, 1985; Miranda-Linne & Melin, 1992; Spradlin & Siegel, 1982). The consensus for the relative value of discrete trial training from these studies (see McGee, Krantz, & McClannahan, 1985 and Miranda-Linne, & Melin, 1992) are those of faster acquisition, and a more efficient and higher frequency of correct responses. The effectiveness of incidental teaching procedures, although slower going during the teaching conditions, increased during the follow up conditions, and even surpassed the effects of discrete trial training. These studies therefore suggest that although incidental teaching procedures may take longer, they may also lead to more perma-nent performance change which is more generalized. These studies, along with the Sundberg and Partington chapter, demonstrate quite clearly that both techniques are valuable, and both should be viewed as complementary methods for facilitating language development. It may be valuable, then, to continue to study the compara-tive effectiveness of these techniques, and given the above-mentioned results, it seems that long term follow up data will be essential in future studies.

There has been some debate in the literature as to which technique to use when. Carr (1983) for example, proposed that nonverbal children with autism must acquire language forms through discrete trial instruction before they can be used in inciden-tal teaching. Halle (1982), suggested an integrative model in which the mand model, delay, and incidental teaching techniques are used sequentially over time. Sundberg and Partington argue quite effectively that "the issue as to which approach is the most effective may not be that simple. Since there is such a wide variation among children with autism, no single approach would probably work for all children."

Sundberg and Partington continue to argue that "a fundamental problem with the different behavioral approaches to language training presented in the literature is that they are not based on a behavioral analysis of language." They remind us in a very eloquent fashion that what needs to be demonstrated is not a comparison of expressive versus receptive language gain, or discrete trial versus natural environ-ment training effects, but rather a return to a definition of language deficits and remediation based on Skinner's initial analysis of verbal behavior. They argue that we need to examine both approaches in relation to Skinner's analysis of verbal behavior as a conceptual framework of language. Sundberg and Partington provide a thorough analysis of each training approach, examining in detail the advantages and disadvantages of both instructional techniques. One minor disagreement with their analysis, however, could be that they, like many others, suggest that a disad-vantage of discrete trial training is its use of consequences irrelevant to the response (e.g., delivery of an M&M for correct labeling of a ball). Whereas they suggest that the natural environment training milieu would provide a possibly more relevant reinforcer (access to ball playing in this example), an alternative suggestion is that any technique will have used relevant consequences if they in fact prove to be the most effective.

Sundberg and Partington also remind us that both discrete trial and natural environment techniques involve receptive and expressive language training. Skinner's (1957) analysis of verbal behavior would indicate that discrete trial training primarily trains tacts, while natural environment training is primarily the training of mands. Sundberg and Partington suggest that both are effective procedures, and each offers specific advantages for teaching certain types of verbal behavior. They remind us that it may be counter-productive to continue to debate as to which training technique is more effective. Rather, we should concentrate on what both techniques have to offer to language acquisition (via a rigorous analysis of verbal behavior), and how effectively to combine both techniques for any individual client.

In clinical practice it becomes quickly apparent that no two autistic children are the same, and therefore, no two children follow an identical learning path. For many children there is no easy answer as to how much training should to be implemented in a discrete trial versus a natural environment format. The learning path for each child is individual and transient at any given moment in his or her training regime. The balance of the approaches will change across time for any given child, and the predominance of one technique over another is a continuously present clinical judgement that involves many factors and processes. I have often found that with many very young children (i.e. 18-24 months old) it is more appropriate to begin therapy with a predominance of natural language training, whereas strategies for older children often involve shaping the natural language process. In some cases, it may be necessary to achieve appropriate focusing and attention from the child before the child can reap the benefits of the natural language approach. I often find that I need to work on attention and focusing at table top type activities before I can direct the child's attention to an object a few feet away, then across the room, then from another room or anywhere in the natural environment. This is in accordance with Sundberg and Partington's argument, as they note that it is most important to consider the existing skills of the individual child when determining the best approach for his individual language needs. They suggest that the balance between discrete trail training and natural environment training may change frequently during the language acquisition process, but that training should always include both approaches.

Given the above analysis, it seems contradictory that Sundberg and Partington end their chapter by suggesting five general phases which would be appropriate for combining discrete trial training and natural language training during the language acquisition process. Although they acknowledge that these five phases may need blending and overlapping, I find it difficult to try to fit any two clinical cases into the same pattern of combining techniques. I do however, applaud the attempt to (a) consider that both techniques need to be combined during each phase, and (b) that overlapping and blending are necessary to benefit different children's individual, and highly variable, language acquisition processes.

When examining the language acquisition process through Skinner's analysis of verbal behavior, Sundberg and Partington vividly remind us to return to looking at the individual child's verbal behavior problems. This point is paramount in the chapter, and it raises the fact that all behavioral support programs, be they decelerative or accelerative (i.e. language acquisition programs) programming, are subject to the goodness-of-fit framework projected by Bailey (1990). Bailey suggested this framework in guiding their family-focused early intervention approach to describe the suitability of the match between early intervention support and the unique characteristics of children and their families. In addition, Albin et al. (1995) emphasized that all behavioral support plans must not only be technically sound, but need also to fit well with the people and the environments where implementation occurs. I submit that language acquisition plans should also fit these criteria. All clinicians have had the experience of designing very elegant and technically sound programs that are: (1) poorly and inconsistently implemented, (2) implemented but not maintained across significant time periods, or (3) simply collect dust in a desk drawer without ever being utilized. Unless our plans are individualized and take into account all of the various aspects of each child's environment and support people, we may be setting ourselves up for unrealistic expectations. Therefore, it may be impossible to categorize all language acquisition programs into the five phases that Sundberg and Partington are suggesting.

When trying to facilitate natural language training with children, much of the training encompasses play skills. I therefore suggest in preparing for this technique that we not only study the behavioral literature (i.e. Strain et al. 1985), but that we may also find value in the literature of other professionals (e.g., Wolfberg, 1995) in enhancing children's play skills. Wolfberg provides some very interesting analyses of the developmental stages of play skills, and provides some useful points for enhancing one's role as a facilitator to engage social interaction, communication, and play skills while developing appropriate peer mediated interactions.

Additionally, when trying to implement natural environment training with nonverbal children, a clinician could run into some obstacles. For example, it may be very difficult as a facilitator to attend to, and get attention from, the child in the natural environment when using sign language. One should examine some of Sundberg and Partington's other work in (a) using Skinner's 1957 analysis of verbal behavior to examine appropriate response options for nonverbal persons (1993) and (b) the difficulty of a child who uses sign language to acquire a tact repertoire (1994). In this study they demonstrated that the verbal stimuli blocked the establishment of stimulus control from nonverbal to verbal stimuli. This may give rise to some functional difficulties when trying to implement natural environment training with nonverbal children. Can we as the facilitators use nonverbal stimuli to avoid stimulus blocking, and still maintain focusing and attention when traveling around the natural environment? In this case, it may be easier and more effective to begin the language training process in the discrete trial format rather than in the natural environment training format.

Overall, we must commend Sundberg and Partington for this eloquent chapter which prompts clinicians to return to the basics in the dilemmas of language training. Sundberg and Partington postulate in this chapter that "a fundamental problem with the different behavioral approaches to language training presented in the literature . . . is that they are not based on a behavioral analysis of language." Sundberg and Partington remind us in this chapter that what needs to be demonstrated is not a battle of expressive versus receptive learning or discrete trial versus natural environment training, but rather a return to a definition of language deficits and remediation based on Skinner's initial analysis of verbal behavior. They very effectively examine both approaches in relation to Skinner's analysis of verbal behavior as a conceptual framework of language.

References

Albin, R.W., Lucyshyn, J.M., Horner, R.H., & Flannery, K.B. (1996). Contextual fit for behavioral support plans: A model for "goodness of fit." In L.K. Keogel, R.L. Keogel, & G. Dunlap (Eds.), *Positive behavioral support: Including people with difficult behavior in the community* (pp. 81-98). Baltimore: Paul H. Brookes.

Baer, D. M., & Guess, D. (1971). Receptive training of adjectival inflections in mental retardates. *Journal of Applied Behavior Analysis, 4,* 129-139.

Baer, D. M., & Sherman, J. A. (1964). Reinforcement of generalized imitation in young children. *Journal of Experimental Child Psychology, 1,* 37-49.

Bailey, D. B., Simeonson, R. J., Winton, P. J., Huntington, G. S., Comfort, M., Isbell, P., O'Donnell, K. J., & Helm, J. M. (1990). Family-focused intervention: A functional model for planning, implementing, and evaluating individualized family services in early intervention. *Journal of the Division for Early Childhood, 10,* 156-171.

Brackbill, Y. (1958). Extinction of the smiling response in infants as a function of reinforcement schedule. *Child Development, 29,* 115-124.

Campbell, C. R. & Stremel-Campbell, K. (1982). Programming "loose training" as a strategy to facilitate language generalization. *Journal of Applied Behavior Analysis, 15,* 295-301.

Carr, E. G. (1983). Behavioral approaches to language and communication. In E. Schopler & G. Mesibov (Eds.), *Current issues in autism, volume III: Communication problems in autism* (pp.37-57). New York: Plenum.

Dunlap, G. (1984). The influence of task variation and maintenance tasks on the learning and effect of autistic children. *Journal of Experimental Child Psychology, 37,* 41-46.

Eisenberg, L. & Kanner, L. (1956). Early infantile autism: 1943-1955. *American Journal of Orthopsychiatry, 26,* 55-65.

Elliott, R.O. Jr., Hall, K., & Soper, H.V. (1991). Analog language teaching versus natural language teaching: Generalization and retention of language learning for adults with autism and mental retardation. *Journal of Autism and Developmental Disorders, 21,* 433-447.

Faw, G. D., Reid, D. H., Schepis, M. N., Fitzgerald, J. R., & Welty, P. A. (1981). Involving institutional staff in the development and maintenance of sign language skills with profoundly retarded persons. *Journal of Applied Behavior Analysis, 14,* 411-423.

Goetz, L., Gee, K., & Sailor, W. (1985). Using a behavioral chain interruption strategy to teach communication skills to students with severe disabilities. *Journal of the Association for Persons with Severe Handicaps, 10,* 21-30.

Green, G. (1996). What does research tell us? In C. Maurice, G. Green and S. C. Luce (Eds.), *Behavioral intervention for young children with autism. A manual for parents and professionals.* (pp.29-44). Texas: Pro-ed.

Greenspoon, J. (1955). The reinforcing effect of two spoken sounds on the frequency of two responses. *American Journal of Psychology, 68,* 409-416.

Guess, S., Sailor, W., Rutherford, G., & Baer, D. M. (1968). An experimental analysis of linguistic development: The productive use of the plural morpheme. *Journal of Applied Behavior Analysis, 1,* 297-306.

Halle, J.W., Marshall, A. M., & Spradlin, J. (1981). Time delay: A technique to increase language use and facilitate generalization in retarded children. *Journal of Applied Behavior Analysis, 12,* 431-439.

Hart, B. M. & Risley, T. R. (1968). Establishing use of descriptive adjectives in the spontaneous speech of disadvantaged preschool children. *Journal of Applied Behavior Analysis, 8,* 411-420.

Hart, B. M. & Risley, T. R. (1980). In vivo language intervention: Unanticipated general effects. *Journal of Applied Behavior Analysis, 13,* 407-432.

Haugan, G. M., & McIntire, R. W. (1972). Comparison of vocal, imitation, tactile stimulation, and food as reinforcers for infant vocalizations. *Developmental Psychology, 6,* 201-209.

Israel, A. C. (1978). Some thoughts on correspondence between saying and doing. *Journal of Applied Behavior Analysis, 11,* 271-276.

Keller, M. F., & Bucher, B. D. (1979). Transfer between receptive and productive language in developmentally disabled children. *Journal of Applied Behavior Analysis, 12,* 311.

Keogel, R.L., O'Dell, M.C., & Keogel, L.K. (1987). A natural language teaching paradigm for nonverbal autistic children. *Journal of Autism and Developmental Disorders, 17,* 187-200.

Lovaas, O. I. (1987). Behavioral treatment and normal educational and intellectual functioning in young autistic children. *Journal of Consulting and Clinical Psychology, 55,* 3-9.

Lovass, O. I. & Smith, T. (1988). Intensive behavioral treatment for young autistic children. In B. B. Lahey & A. E. Kazdin (Eds.), *Advances in clinical child psychology* (Vol. 11, 285-324) New York: Plenum.

McGee, G. G., Krantz, P. J., & McClannahan, L. E. (1985). The facilitative effects of incidental teaching on preposition use by autistic children. *Journal of Applied Behavior Analysis, 18,* 17-31.

Michael, J. L. (1984). Verbal behavior. *Journal of the Experimental Analysis of Behavior, 42,* 363-376.

Michael, J. L. (1988). Establishing operations and the mand. *The Analysis of Verbal Behavior, 3,* 3-9.

Miranda-Linne, F., & Melin, L. (1992). Acquisition, generalization, and spontaneous use of color adjectives: A comparison of incidental teaching and traditional discrete trial procedures for children with autism. *Research in Developmental Disabilities, 13*, 191-210.

Neef, N. A., Walters, J., & Egel, A. L. (1984). Establishing generative yes/no responses in developmentally disabled children. *Journal of Applied Behavior Analysis, 17*, 453-460.

Oah, S., & Dickinson, A. M. (1989). A review of empirical studies of verbal behavior. *The Analysis of Verbal Behavior, 7*, 53-68.

Osgood, C. E. (1958). *Verbal Behavior*, by B. F. Skinner. *Contemporary Psychology, 3*, 212-214.

Partington, J. W., Sundberg, M. L., Newhouse, L., & Spengler, S. M. (1994). Overcoming an autistic child's failure to acquire a tact repertoire. Special issue: Integrating basic and applied research. *Journal of Applied Behavior Analysis, 27*, 733-734.

Peterson, R. F. (1968). Imitation: A basic behavioral mechanism. In H. N. Sloane, Jr., and B. D. MacAulay (Eds.), *Operant procedures in remedial speech and language training* (pp. 61-74). Boston: Houghton Mifflin.

Pierce, K.L. & Schreibman, L. (1994). Teaching daily living skills to children with autism in unsupervised settings through pictorial self-management. *Journal of Applied Behavior Analysis, 27*, 471-481.

Rheingold, H. L., Gewirtz, J. L., & Ross, H. W. (1959). Social conditioning of vocalizations in the infant. *Journal of Comparative and Physiological Psychology, 52*, 68-73.

Routh, D. K. (1969). Conditioning of vocal response differentiation in infants. *Developmental Psychology, 1*, 219-226.

Rutter, M. (1968). Concepts of autism: A review of research. *Journal of Child Psychology and Psychiatry, 9*, 1-25.

Sailor, W., & Taman, T. (1972). Stimulus factors in the training of prepositional usage in three autistic children. *Journal of Applied Behavior Analysis, 5*, 183-190.

Schreibman, L. (1988*). Autism*. California: Sage.

Skinner, B. F. (1938). *The behavior of organisms*. New York: Appleton-Century-Crofts.

Skinner, B. F. (1957). *Verbal behavior*. New York: Appleton-Century-Crofts.

Smith, R., Michael, J., & Sundberg, M. (1995). Automatic reinforcement and automatic punishment in infant vocal behavior. *Analysis of Verbal Behavior, 13*, 39-48.

Spradlin, J., & Siegel, G. (1982). Language training in natural and clinical environments. *Journal of Speech and Hearing Disorders, 47*, 2-6.

Strain, P.S., Hoyson, M., & Jamieson, B. (1985). Normally developing preschoolers as intervention agents for autistic-like children: Effects on class deportment and social interaction. *Journal of the Division for Early Childhood, 9*, 105-115.

Sundberg, M. L., & Partington, J. W. (1993). Selecting a response form for nonverbal persons: Facilitated communication, pointing systems, or sign language? *Analysis of Verbal Behavior, 11*, 99-116.

Taylor, B. A. & Harris, S. L. (1995). Teaching children with autism to seek information: Acquisition of novel information and generalization of responding. *Journal of Applied Behavior Analysis, 28,* 3-14.

Todd, G. A., & Palmer, B. (1968). Social reinforcement of infant babbling. *Child Development, 39,* 591-596.

Weisberg, P. (1963). Social and nonsocial conditioning of infant vocalizations. *Child Development, 34,* 377-388.

Wolfberg, P. J. (1995) Enhancing children's play. In K. A. Quill (Ed.), *Teaching children with autism: Strategies to enhance communication and socialization,* (pp.193-218). New York: Delmar.

Young, J. M., Krantz, P. J., McClannahan, L. E., & Poulson, C. L. (1994). Generalized imitation and response-class formation in children with autism. *Journal of Applied Behavior Analysis, 27,* 685-697.

Chapter 8

Naturalistic Teaching Strategies for Acquisition, Generalization, and Maintenance of Speech in Children With Autism

Marjorie H. Charlop-Christy and Linda A. LeBlanc
Claremont McKenna College

One of the most enduring obstacles in the treatment of children with autism is their pervasive failure to develop functional speech (Charlop & Haymes, 1994). Not only is speech acquisition difficult, but there are continued problems with maintenance and generalization once speech is taught (Schreibman, 1988). Naturalistic teaching strategies emerged out of the need to facilitate speech acquisition and promote generalization in natural environments such as in the home, school, and community (Halle, 1984; Halle, Baer, & Spradlin, 1981). In general, naturalistic teaching strategies incorporate three vital elements: (a) motivation enhancing techniques, (b) functional relationships, and (c) variables that facilitate generalization.

The motivation enhancing techniques include strategies such as varied reinforcers, child choice, and repeated preference assessments with preferred stimuli and novel stimuli to indicate which items are currently of interest (DeLeon & Iwata, 1996; Egel, 1981). In addition, motivation is enhanced by incorporating therapy environments that are less structured and associated with play. Second, functional relationships are established between spoken words and access to reinforcing events, thus maximizing the motivational effects of existing establishing operations and establishing mands as a response class (Michael, 1993). Finally, naturalistic teaching strategies include variables that facilitate generalization, such as less structured teaching settings (free play), incorporation of natural environments (home) as teaching environments, the use of parents, teachers, and others who co-occupy the natural environment, and use of natural reinforcers and intermittent contingencies (c.f. Stokes & Baer, 1977).

Naturalistic teaching strategies are a departure from early discrete trial speech training approaches (e.g., Lovaas, 1981) in several aspects. First, naturalistic teaching strategies focus on natural speech production rather than on rote memorization of speech phrases and drills of facts and responses. Second, naturalistic teaching strategies provide a more motivating, enjoyable work environment for children, and focus on speech that is more likely to generalize (Schreibman & Charlop-Christy, in press). Data indicate that naturalistic teaching strategies are associated with rapid behavior gains (e.g., Charlop, Schreibman, & Thibodeau, 1985), generalized treatment effects (Schreibman & Koegel, in press), and positive attitudes on behalf of behavior change agents (Schreibman, Kaneko, & Koegel, 1991).

Below is a brief discussion of the literature on the three components of naturalistic teaching strategies: motivation, functional relationships, and generalization and maintenance. Also included in this chapter is a presentation of several naturalistic teaching strategies researched at the Claremont Autism Center. There are many other naturalistic teaching strategies, such as incidental teaching (e.g., Hart & Risley, 1975; McGee, Krantz, & McClannahan, 1985), milieu therapy (Rogers-Warren & Warren, 1980), and pivotal response training (Koegel et al., 1989), that have influenced the development of our procedures or that were researched concurrently. However, the purpose of this chapter is to highlight those that we have been developing at the Claremont Autism Center over the past 14 years.

Motivation

Children with autism are frequently not motivated by the same social reinforcers that motivate typical children (e.g., achievement, praise, success). All too often, the therapy or teaching setting is associated with a lack of reinforcers and the presence of aversive stimuli such as difficult tasks (Schreibman & Charlop-Christy, in press). Children with autism will frequently try to escape the aversive work setting by engaging in inappropriate behaviors such as tantrums and self-injurious behavior (Carr, 1977). Thus, increasing motivation to work on difficult tasks is crucial to the child's continued improvement, and to overall treatment success. The importance of motivation is clearly reflected in the number of published studies which have addressed strategies to increase motivation to learn for children with autism.

One line of research has focused on interspersing trials of previously learned "maintenance" tasks with trials of new "acquisition" tasks. Dunlap and Koegel (1980) demonstrated that trial interspersal was associated with increased attempts to respond and fewer avoidance and escape behaviors, which may be indicators of superior motivation. Charlop, Kurtz and Milstein, (1993) expanded upon this evidence by noting that the presentation of maintenance tasks is important, but the schedule of reinforcement for both maintenance tasks and acquisition tasks is perhaps more important. Since few correct responses are typically made during the initial learning of a task, procedures that include the interspersal of maintenance tasks ensure that the child maintains a relatively high density of reinforcement even when he is not successful with the new task.

Another research approach to this motivation problem is the identification of new reinforcers. Charlop, Kurtz, and Casey (1990) assessed the effectiveness of using autistic children's aberrant behaviors as reinforcers to increase appropriate responding. In a series of three experiments, reinforcer conditions of self-stimulation, delayed echolalia, and obsessive behaviors were compared with food reinforcers and varied (i.e., food/aberrant behavior) reinforcer conditions. For example, during sessions of the delayed echolalia condition each child was permitted to utter a favored delayed echo (e.g., say "Eat your beef stew"). During sessions with self-stimulation as a reinforcer, the child was allowed to engage in 5 seconds of an idiosyncratic stereotypy (e.g., tap his hand for 5 seconds). Finally, in sessions that employed objects of obsession as a reinforcer the child could have brief access to an object with which he/she was preoccupied (e.g., look at a Honda Civic catalog for 5 seconds). The results of these three experiments suggested that these aberrant behaviors could be easily controlled and used effectively as reinforcers for new behaviors, without increasing the free operant frequencies of aberrant behaviors. The premise of using aberrant behaviors as reinforcers has also been demonstrated to be effective in reducing inappropriate behaviors by allowing access to the item of obsession contingent upon periods of nonoccurrence of inappropriate behaviors (Charlop-Christy & Haymes, 1996). Finally, a comparison of token economies using tokens with no previously assessed value and tokens deemed objects of obsession has suggested that token reinforcers are more effective if they are items of obsession (Charlop-Christy & Haymes, in press).

Functional Relationships

The functional relationship between inappropriate behaviors and reinforcing events was documented in the literature before functional relationships were incorporated into speech training (Carr, 1977; Iwata, Dorsey, Slifer, Bauman, & Richman, 1982/1994). The use of functional relationships between speech and its outcome (reinforcer) has been examined more recently in the literature on incidental teaching and milieu therapy with children with autism (McGee et al., 1985; Rogers-Warren & Warren, 1980). The naturalistic teaching strategies discussed later in this chapter will elaborate upon the necessity of the functional relationship between a verbal utterance and a related reinforcer, as opposed to the relationship between a verbal utterance and an arbitrary or unrelated event, such as food. It is important to note that while food reinforcers are often functionally related to verbal behavior (e.g., "I want chips"; Charlop et al., 1985), food may not be functionally related when a child requests a toy (e.g., "train") or when the child imitates a verbal model.

Other studies have confirmed the importance of a functional relationship between a verbal behavior and the subsequent reinforcing event. For example, Koegel, O'Dell, and Koegel (1987) demonstrated that appropriate social behaviors might be increased by allowing the child to choose the task or activity and potential reinforcer. This emphasis on choice facilitates functional relationships by maximizing the potential effects of establishing operations as motivation for mands (Michael, 1982). Additionally, shaping, or the reinforcement of successive approximations to correct responses, allows the reinforcer to be presented much earlier in the acquisition process and on a denser schedule (Laski, Charlop, & Schreibman, 1988). Thus, the connection between behavior and natural reinforcer is more likely due to a greater number of successful trials (Koegel, O'Dell, & Dunlap, 1988).

Carr, Binkoff, Kologinsky, and Eddy (1978) taught children with autism to use sign language to request items that were likely to be found in the natural environment. The children were taught spontaneously to request (via signing) their favorite toys, as opposed to specific educational stimuli found only in the training environment. This training led to generalized spontaneous signing. One can see the importance of the functional relationship component of naturalistic teaching strategies in terms of acquisition of speech behaviors, and in relation to motivation (discussed above) and generalization (discussed below).

Generalization and Maintenance

The acquisition of speech or any other behavior is meaningless unless generalization and maintenance occur over time. Thus, naturalistic teaching strategies incorporate many of the provisions for facilitating generalization and maintenance that were outlined in the seminal article by Stokes and Baer (1977). One approach to facilitating generalization is to make the treatment environment more similar to the natural environment. This similarity can be promoted in several ways. First, the use of intermittent reinforcement schedules during treatment provides a learning environment that more closely approximates the contingencies in effect in the natural environment. Several studies have suggested that the use of intermittent schedules increases the durability of treatment gains by reducing the discriminability of the reinforcement schedules used in treatment and non-treatment settings (Charlop et al., 1993; Koegel & Rincover, 1977). As will be described later, naturalistic teaching strategies also incorporate play settings, which facilitate the transition to and similarity with the natural environment (Charlop-Christy & Carpenter, 1997, October; Laski et al., 1988; Valdez, 1998).

Naturalistic teaching strategies also incorporate procedures that provide direct skill training in the settings in which generalization needs to occur (referred to as sequential modification by Stokes and Baer, 1977). However, the impracticality of training a behavior in every potential situation frequently necessitates the use of an alternative approach (i.e., training multiple exemplars; Stokes & Baer). This technique may also be difficult because it is usually impossible to determine beforehand the necessary number of situations or exemplars that will be required before generalization is achieved. However, much success with this approach has been reported in the literature (e.g., Laski et al., 1988).

Stokes and Baer (1977) also suggested using mediated generalization. This procedure focuses on teaching a target response that is likely to occur in both treatment and nontreatment situations. The most common mediator is language. Children giving self-instructions in different environments are using this generalization strategy. Few studies have addressed the use of mediated generalization with children with autism. Charlop (1983) demonstrated that children with autism might be able to use their echolalia as a verbal mediator. Self-management procedures may also be considered mediated generalization because the target behavior (self-management) can be taken along from the training environment to other settings (e.g.,

Koegel & Koegel, 1986; Pierce & Schreibman, 1995; Stahmer, 1995). It is clear that research into achieving generalization of treatment effects has become a top priority for naturalistic teaching strategies.

Naturalistic Teaching Strategies

Now that we have presented a definition of naturalistic teaching strategies and provided a brief discussion of the literature in the three main aspects of naturalistic teaching strategies, we will provide a brief presentation of selected strategies. As stressed earlier, the examples presented are strategies that are being researched at the Claremont Autism Center. These strategies are a few of the ones that we use, in conjunction with many other procedures in our treatment of children with autism. In addition, many other researchers have developed a number of intriguing approaches to the study and use of naturalistic teaching strategies, but unfortunately are not in the immediate purview of this chapter.

Natural Language Paradigm

The Natural Language Paradigm (NLP) was designed to combine aspects of discrete trial language-based programs (e.g., Lovaas, Koegel, Simmons, & Stevens-Long, 1973) with naturalistic programs, such as the mand-model procedure (Rogers-Warren & Warren, 1980). NLP was originally designed by Koegel et al. (1987) and expanded upon by Laski. et al. (1988). NLP is a play-oriented speech and language training program which is used frequently at the Claremont Autism Center, both to teach speech to non-verbal children, and to improve speech with children with some verbal abilities (e.g., echolalia). As you will see below, a motivation-oriented procedure makes work on a difficult-to-teach behavior (e.g., speech) fun for both the child and the therapist.

There are four basic components of NLP. The first is direct reinforcement of verbal attempts. The therapist models a brief verbalization for the child, such as "frog hops," but the child does not need to say the entire phrase in order to receive reinforcers. The child may make an attempt, such as "fro" or "hop." The reinforcement consists of praise and access to the object used in the demonstration. Shaping increases motivation by maximizing the likelihood of the child's success while the use of natural reinforcers enhances functional relationships and generalization.

The second component is turn taking with the toys. Both the therapist and the child take turns talking about and playing with the toy. First, the therapist models a verbalization about the toy. When the child either imitates the verbalization or makes his attempt to imitate, the therapist gives the child the toy for a few seconds for "his turn." Then it is the therapist's turn again, and she takes the toys and models another phrase about the toy. This turn-taking process facilitates generalization by increasing the similarity between the NLP sessions and the natural environment. In addition, turn taking adds a more game-like or play atmosphere to the work session which may facilitate motivation. Although not yet directly measured, it is possible that the turn-taking component of NLP will also facilitate social behavior by directly teaching an important and developmentally appropriate social skill.

The third basic component to NLP is task variation and the use of multiple exemplars. NLP uses a variety of toys to illustrate a particular phrase, and uses a variety of phrases to describe a particular toy. For example, the therapist can model "frog hops" but then would also model " bunny hops" while demonstrating the hopping movement with the toys. Additionally, the therapist may say "frog hops" for the frog toy, but also vary the phrase and say "frog jumps" or "frog is green." This variation not only makes the speech training session more fun, but also promotes generalization.

Finally, the fourth component is shared control. At the start of each NLP trial, the child selects, from a presented assortment, which toy he would like to play with/speak about. Therefore, the child shares in the control of what is going to be learned in the NLP session. In addition, if the child changes a verbalization or indicates that he would like to play with another object, the therapist should follow the child's lead. For example, if the therapist says "open door" to the dollhouse and the child responds with "go in door" the therapist should pick up the child's lead and then reiterate "go in door." Thus, NLP makes use of the concept of shared control to maximize the effects of momentary changes in establishing operations that may work to increase reinforcer effectiveness.

You can get the "feel" for an NLP session from the above four essential components. NLP is a more relaxed, less structured way to teach speech using a play (i.e., sharing, turn-taking) approach. Not only is motivation higher, but parents report that they enjoy this way of working at home with their child better than discrete trial methods. The general procedural steps for NLP are described below. For more detailed information see Charlop-Christy and Kelso (1997), Koegel et al. (1987), or Laski et al. (1988).

NLP Procedural Steps

1. Sit facing the child either in child-sized chairs or on the floor. Provide an assortment of toys, books, and functional objects (e.g., toothbrushes, cups). These items should be of interest to the child and be placed adjacent to you, but out of the child's immediate reach.
2. Place three toys/objects in front of the child and ask him to choose one. The child may indicate his choice by pointing, reaching, or saying the name of the object. Initially, you may need to prompt the child to make a selection.
3. Retain the chosen item and remove the others.
4. Repeatedly model an appropriate phrase while engaging in the corresponding activity. If the child chose a toy car, you might say "roll car" while rolling the car back and forth.
5. Pause for 5 seconds to allow the child verbally to imitate, or to attempt to imitate, by making an approximation of the modeled verbalization. Initially, nonverbal children may utter any sound in order to gain access to the toy. In our example, the therapist says "roll car" while rolling the car. She pauses to allow the child to imitate, echo, or approximate the model. The child

responds with "ah." If that response is appropriate for that child, the therapist should then provide praise (e.g., "good talking" or "good try") and give the child the car. Clearly, "ah" would not be an acceptable response if the child had previously said "car" many times.

6. If necessary, prompt the child to speak by allowing the child to have his hand on the toy with your hand over the child's hand. Do not let go of the toy until the child makes his attempt to verbalize. Remove your hand and release the toy to the child contingent upon a verbalization. This provides the child with immediate and direct reinforcement.

7. As the child plays with the object, the therapist should repeat the modeled phrase a few times. For example, while the child is rolling the car, the therapist says "roll car, roll car, roll car."

8. After the child plays with the toy for 3-5 seconds, say "my turn" and have the child give you the toy. Model a different phrase for the same object (e.g., "drive car" or "car goes fast").

9. After a few exchanges between therapist and child with a few different modeled verbalizations, the child should select a new toy. Choose 3 other toys from the adjacent assortment and ask the child to choose. Repeat steps 4-8 with this new object. After several toys have been played with, you may take a break or go on to a different task.

10. Remember to change activities and words frequently to maintain the child's interest.

The NLP was designed to combine aspects of discrete trial language-based programs (e.g., one-on-one training sessions) with aspects of incidental programs (e.g., shared control). The procedure was designed to address the perceived trade-off between the tight stimulus control employed in traditional discrete trial programs with looser stimulus control employed in incidental programs. Initially, researchers expected that tighter stimulus control resulted in much faster acquisition but poor generalization, while very loosely structured programs resulted in much slower acquisition. Our data suggest that generalization is promoted with NLP while rapid acquisition is maintained.

For example, Laski et al. (1988) evaluated the effectiveness of NLP when used by parents of two groups of children with autism ("mute" and echolalic children). In this study, parents were trained to criterion on program implementation in a clinic setting, but all treatment sessions between parent and child occurred in the home. The results indicated that the children's speech increased quite rapidly. The most speech gains were seen with the echolalic children. However, the "mute" children also improved dramatically. It is important to keep in mind that during baseline the children were receiving discrete-trial speech training as described by Lovaas (1981), but failed to learn this way. NLP was thus associated with rapid learning and speech gains that generalized to untrained settings. Parents reported that they enjoyed the NLP sessions, and that they thought their children had enjoyed the sessions as well. While the motivation effects were not directly measured, the results of this study suggested that NLP is an appropriate naturalistic teaching strategy for both "mute" and echolalic children, and that parents can successfully be used as trainers.

Speech and Play Enhancement for Autistic Kids (SPEAK)

While NLP presents trials in a play-oriented manner, it is clear that the concept of "trials" is still in place, and that the loose structure of a free-play environment is not used. NLP may be seen as the first step in the direction of loosening of structure and using a therapy setting that more closely approximates a play situation. Speech Play Enhancement for Autistic Kids (SPEAK) was designed to integrate training for both speech and play in young children with autism. Incorporating speech training into a play setting can create a more enjoyable learning environment by enhancing child motivation, while allowing the therapist to teach two appropriate target behaviors (play skills and speech).

Importantly, the SPEAK program maximizes the effects of natural developmental skill progression which is evident in typical children, and may be evident in children with autism. It is well documented that typical children learn to play as early as infancy, well before they learn to speak (Nelson, 1973). Indeed, while conducting a program evaluation study of the Claremont Autism Center, Kelso and Charlop-Christy (1996, May) found that children with autism under the age of 6 years made more gains in play skills, while their older counterparts (6 years and older) demonstrated more gains in speech. Thus, play behaviors and speech may be developmentally related in children with autism, with gains in play behaviors occurring before speech gains. The SPEAK program attempts to capitalize on this possible developmental progression and to "piggyback" the acquisition of the more difficult behavior (speech) on the easier gains seen with a higher probability behavior (play). Development of such a naturalistic teaching strategy seems quite appropriate since (a) it may be developmentally appropriate to incorporate play, (b) play is easier to teach than speech, and finally (c) play behavior is an appropriate target in and of itself.

The SPEAK program is conducted in a free-play setting with preferred toys, including items with which the child may be obsessed. The free-play setting more closely approximates the natural environment and, therefore, facilitates generalization. In addition, a free-play setting is more likely to contain varied reinforcers that may motivate the child. The use of preferred toys, especially the use of toys that may be the objects of obsession, may further maximize the motivating features of the learning environment (Charlop et al., 1990). Also, these kinds of items available in a free-play setting are more likely to be encountered in the natural environment and may promote generalization.

The child and the trainer initially play independently, and the child is allowed to choose any toy and move from item to item according to changing preferences. This "child choice" is considered an important component of SPEAK which allows the child to indicate changes in preference which may affect reinforcer effectiveness. Approximately each minute, a "contact" occurs in which the therapist models a contextually appropriate speech utterance. The speech utterance is a phrase or word about the item in the child's possession. For example, if the child were playing with a puzzle, "in" would be appropriate to the activity. The label of the item may also be modeled for the child to imitate and/or approximate. For example, the therapist could merely say "ball" when the child is playing with the ball. Any approximation would be reinforced with (a) access to the item (giving the ball to the child), (b) access to an enjoyable play activity (making a basket with the ball), (c) praise ("good job"), and (d) a natural response by the therapist ("I like the ball, too"). If the child does not have a toy at the time of the "contact", the trainer would suggest one and model both appropriate play and speech. At each contact, if the child was not playing appropriately, both play and speech would be modeled by the trainer but no reprimands would be presented for inappropriate manipulation of the item.

In a recent investigation, Valdez (1998) demonstrated that the SPEAK program could be used to increase both play and speech in three young boys with autism who participated in the after-school program at the Claremont Autism Center. A multiple baseline design across participants was used to evaluate the effectiveness of the SPEAK program with two children who demonstrated no speech in baseline and one child who demonstrated low frequencies of speech in baseline. This latter participant merely iterated letters of the alphabet and numbers out of context. During baseline, a therapist was instructed to talk and play with the child for 10 minutes in a free play setting. In addition, identical baseline generalization probes were conducted with unfamiliar persons. Treatment sessions consisting of the SPEAK program were alternated with generalization probes with the naive participant from the baseline condition. SPEAK was effective in increasing speech in all three children, and all three children demonstrated increases in appropriate play. Perhaps the most important finding was that both speech and play generalized across persons and settings.

Multiple Incidental Teaching Sessions (MITS)

A third naturalistic teaching strategy recently developed at the Claremont Autism Center is Multiple Incidental Teaching Sessions (MITS). MITS represents a compromise between traditional incidental teaching and discrete trial procedures. MITS incorporates the assumptions of incidental teaching by conducting training in the natural environment using naturally occurring opportunities and situation-appropriate functional phrases (McGee et al., 1985). In this manner, MITS is easy for parents to learn and conduct in their home. In addition, MITS incorporates additional training trials commonly used in discrete trial procedures to maximize the likelihood of rapid response acquisition, which is commonly associated with discrete trial training procedures (e.g., Lovaas, 1981).

In the MITS procedure, the child initiates the interaction in the natural setting much like incidental teaching procedures. However, like milieu therapy, the parent controls the number of daily trials by incorporating practice trials (Rogers-Warren & Warren, 1980). For example, the child may initiate the interaction by approaching a closed door, allowing a training opportunity for the phrase "open door." The parent can then conduct the first trial by (a) providing a brief time delay to allow the opportunity for spontaneous speech to occur, (b) modeling the phrase if no spontaneous speech occurs, (c) praising/reinforcing an appropriate verbal approximation, and (d) conducting two immediate additional practice trials. The practice trials might be conducted by having the parent respond to the first verbal attempt with praise and the prompt "Let's practice that again." Thus, three training trials are conducted in each block: the initial trial and two practice trials. Typically, two training blocks of three trials are conducted throughout the day.

Parents have reported satisfaction with the MITS procedure for several reasons. First, the MITS procedure is easy for parents to learn and to implement in a natural setting. Second, MITS is preferred by parents because they can determine which training opportunities they will use for training in accordance with their daily schedule. Structured massed training trials may be too cumbersome to fit into a hectic schedule, but two extra practice trials can easily be inserted into regular daily activities. The ease of the procedure and the integration of the procedure into a daily schedule may increase parental implementation of the procedure.

In a recent study, Charlop-Christy and Carpenter (October, 1997) directly compared the effects of incidental teaching, discrete trial teaching, and MITS for speech acquisition and generalization in young children with autism. A multiple baseline design across participants was used to evaluate the effectiveness of each procedure for increasing speech, while the procedures were directly compared for each child by incorporating an alternating treatments design (see Table 1). Each procedure was paired with a different phase for each child. All treatment protocols were implemented in the home by parents who were trained to criterion on each treatment procedure. In addition, generalization probes were conducted in novel settings and with novel people (e.g., siblings).

Each of the treatment procedures was effective in increasing some speech behaviors; however, MITS was the only procedure associated with generalization of spontaneous speech. Discrete trial procedures led to rapid acquisition of imitative speech and more moderate increases in spontaneous speech, but these speech gains did not generalize to new settings or persons. Incidental teaching procedures resulted in slower response acquisition of imitative speech, with no increases in spontaneous speech and no generalization. It should be noted that a longer evaluation of the incidental teaching procedure might have resulted in greater acquisition and generalization of speech. The MITS procedure resulted in a rate of speech acquisition that was comparable to discrete trial methods and resulted in generalization effects that surpassed both other training methods. Finally, parents who participated in the study reported that they were likely to implement the MITS program more frequently and more accurately than discrete trial procedures.

Time Delay

The time delay procedure is used to teach spontaneous speech to children with autism (Charlop et al., 1985; Charlop & Trasowech, 1991; Charlop & Walsh, 1986).

Table 1: Summary of Treatment Conditions in Charlop-Christy & Carpenter (1997).

Treatment Condition	Setting	Number of Trials
IT	natural environment, "as it happens"	1
DT	segregated one-on-one therapy session	10
MITS	natural environment, "as it happens"	6*

* 2 naturally occurring opportunities with 2 additional practice trials at each opportunity

Charlop et al. (1985) defined spontaneous speech as speech in the absence of a verbal cue. Thus, a child's response to a verbal cue such as "say hi," "what's your name?" or "what's this?" would not be considered spontaneous. However, a child who says "hi" upon seeing, you or says "I want coke" upon seeing a soda can has emitted a spontaneous response because no verbal prompt or cue occurred. The time delay procedure works very well for a variety of situations and types of spontaneous speech. Table 2 presents a brief, illustrative (not exhaustive) list of several situations appropriate for use of the time delay procedure to occasion spontaneous speech.

There are two types of time delay: graduated and constant. Graduated time delay involves initiating training with no time interval at all between establishment of the child's attention and modeling an appropriate verbalization. Gradually, the time interval between initial establishment of attention and the verbal model is increased. Therefore, if the therapist is trying to teach a child to say "good morning," she initially establishes eye contact with the child and immediately models "good

Table 2. Appropriate Situations For Use of Time Delay.

To request a desired item, "I want juice"
To request a desired setting, "I want playroom"
To request a desired activity, "I want to play outside"
To request a need, "Go potty"
To express a feeling, "I'm tired"
To provide a greeting, "Hi" "Good morning"
To initiate an interaction, "let's play"
To initiate a conversation, "How are you today"

morning" for the child to imitate. When the child reliably imitates the model with no delay to prompt, the therapist increases the interval between establishing eye contact in the setting and modeling "good morning" by 2-second increments until a delay of 10 seconds is reached. The 10-second delay is considered an appropriate amount of time to expect a response to occur. In the "good morning" example, after the child reliably imitated "good morning" with no delay, the adult would establish eye contact with the child and wait 2 seconds to allow the child an opportunity to emit spontaneous speech. If no spontaneous speech occurred in the 2-second interval, the adult would model the phrase "good morning." After reliably responding at the 2-second interval, the therapist may increase the delay to 4 seconds before modeling the phrase.

As the time delay is gradually increased, stimulus control gradually transfers from the adult's modeled phrase to the delay that is provided, and to the specific setting and stimulus conditions associated with the training environment. The time of day, the child's room, and the first entrance into class all become stimulus conditions associated with the phrase "good morning." The essential feature of time delay is the transfer of control of the child's speech to naturally occurring environmental stimuli and conversational pauses. Constant time delay is also designed to transfer stimulus control of the child's speech to environmental cues rather than adult's prompts. However, constant time delay involves implementing the 10-second delay from the initial training trial. The 10-second delay is maintained throughout the remaining trials until training is successful and spontaneous speech occurs within the 10-second interval between initial eye contact and the verbal model.

The choice between graduated time delay and constant time delay should be based on several variables. First, if the child has relatively little spontaneous speech, then graduated time delay should be implemented. Children with more spontaneous speech may benefit from the constant time delay procedure. Second, graduated time delay should be used to teach abstract spontaneous speech or speech that is not tied to an obvious physical referent, such as in the example of "good morning" above. If the response is more concrete, a constant time delay may prove more effective. For example, if a child grabs for a soda can, you can implement a constant time delay procedure. Establish eye contact, hold the can, and wait ten seconds for the child to say, "I want soda" (or model the phrase "I want soda" after the 10-seond delay). Third, while graduated time delay is highly likely to be effective, correct implementation of the procedure is more difficult because it requires a more extensive knowledge of stimulus fading techniques. While there is no one general rule for choosing one of these procedures, we recommend using graduated time delay to teach new or abstract responses and using constant time delay for later, concrete responses. Below are the procedural steps for using time delay in common situations in a child's daily activities.

Time Delay Procedure for Requests of Items: Graduated Time Delay

1. Present a desired item (e.g., toy, snack) by either holding, lifting it in front of the child, or placing it on the table. For example, hold up a favorite book.
2. Establish eye contact with the child.
3. Immediately model the target phrase "I want book" for the child to imitate.
4. Allow no more than 10 seconds after the modeled phrase for the child to respond. If the child imitates the response (says "I want book"), then provide praise and the book. If the child does not imitate the response, then provide verbal feedback ("no, let's try again").
5. Repeat steps 1-4.
6. If imitation does not occur, present this task again later.
7. After 5 consecutive trials of imitation at a zero-second delay to prompt, increase to a 2-second delay.
8. Repeat steps 1-4 with a 2-second delay.
9. If the child imitates your phrase, then provide reinforcement (praise and book) for imitation. However, now the child may speak spontaneously during the 2-second delay, before the modeled response.
10. After the child either imitates or speaks spontaneously on 5 consecutive trials, go on to the 4-second delay. *Note*: Even if the child is still only imitating speech, increase the delay. Data indicate that time delay works even if only imitative speech occurs in the first few delay levels.
11. Continue the procedure until a 10-second delay is reached. If the child is speaking spontaneously by the 4-6 second delay, continue with gradual fading. Do not skip to the 10-second delay. Gradual fading aides in transfer of stimulus control from the presence of the object (book) to the delay in time.
12. Once the child reliably responds within a 10-second delay, spontaneous speech has occurred.

After successful implementation of time delay, stimulus control has been transferred from the verbal model to the physical referent (e.g., book) or the relevant environmental cues (e.g., time of day). Thus, as spontaneous speech increases, the child learns to request many different items he desires or needs in the absence of adults predicting his needs and prompting "what do you want" or "ask for something."

Summary

In the last 15 years, several naturalistic teaching strategies have been developed to promote imitative and spontaneous speech in young children with autism. The naturalistic teaching strategies presented in this chapter share several common features, including the use of loose stimulus control to promote generalization, incorporation of child choice into task and reinforcer selection, and the use of naturally occurring semi-structured or unstructured play settings (see Table 3). These

Table 3. Comparison of Discrete Trial Procedures With Specific Naturalistic Training Programs

Variable	Discrete Trials	Natural Language Paradigm (NPL)	SPEAK	MITS
Number of Trials	10-20	3-6	1-5	6
Trial Selection	Trainer Choice	Child Choice	Child Choice	Setting dependent with elements of child choice
Stimulus Control	Tight	Loose	Loose	Loose
Setting	Artificial work setting	semi-structured or unstructured play	Unstructured play	Incidental or naturally occurring
Reinforcer	Artificial/ unrelated highly preferred edibles	functional (highly preferred toys)	multiple, functional (praise, activities, highly pre-ferred toys)	functional (activity, or item based child's need or desire)

features are in direct contrast to more structured, discrete-trial language training methods.

Extensive empirical evidence exists to support the use of naturalistic teaching strategies with children with autism (Charlop & Trasowech, 1991; Charlop-Christy & Carpenter, 1997, October; Koegel et al., 1987; Laski et al., 1988). In the past, naturalistic teaching strategies may have been underrated in terms of speed of acquisition, but recent data indicated that responses may be acquired at acceptable rates (Charlop-Christy & Carpenter; Halle, Marshall, & Spradlin, 1984; McGee et al., 1985). More importantly, speech generalizes well when naturalistic teaching strategies are used and both children and parents are motivated to use these strategies (Laski et al., 1988; Schreibman et al., 1991).

Naturalistic teaching strategies are well suited for use by parents and siblings because they create an enjoyable work environment and maximize the motivation of the child with autism (Schreibman & Charlop-Christy, in press). Parents prefer these strategies because they are typically easy to learn, implement, and integrate into a hectic daily schedule (Charlop & Trasowech, 1991). The importance of identifying procedures that parents can implement on a frequent and consistent basis has become a recurrent theme in the language acquisition research literature, as is reflected by the growing number of naturalistic interventions that are available.

In summary, there are a number of naturalistic teaching strategies that can be easily and successfully used to teach speech to children with autism. These techniques provide an alternative strategy to older, more structured teaching methods, and can be easily incorporated into existing treatment programs. Additionally, these naturalistic teaching methods can be used either alone, or in combination with more structured training procedures, to create a comprehensive behavioral intervention system that targets both play and speech. These naturalistic strategies are a good indicator of a positive trend among behavioral intervention approaches to concurrently address language deficits, social behaviors, and to integrate family and community systems.

References

Carr, E. G. (1977). The origins of self-injurious behavior: A review of some hypotheses. *Psychological Bulletin, 84,* 800-816.

Carr, E. G., Binkoff, J. A., Kologinsky, E., & Eddy, M. (1978). Acquisition of sign language by autistic children. I. Expressive labeling. *Journal of Applied Behavior Analysis, 11,* 489-501.

Charlop-Christy, M., & Carpenter, M. (1997, October). Modified Incidental Teaching Sessions (MITS): A procedure for parents to increase spontaneous speech in their children with autism. In M. H. Charlop-Christy (Chair), *New techniques to address language acquisition, social behavior, and severe problem behavior in young children with autism.* Symposium conducted at the annual meeting of the Southern California Association of Behavior Analysis, Pasedena, CA.

Charlop, M. H. (1983). The effects of echolalia on acquisition and generalization of receptive labeling in autistic children. *Journal of Applied Behavior Analysis, 16,* 111-126.

Charlop, M. H., & Haymes, L. K. (1994). Speech and language acquisition and intervention: Behavioral approaches. In J. L. Matson (Ed.), *Autism in children and adults: Etiology, assessment, and intervention* (pp. 213-240). Pacific Grove, CA: Brookes/Cole.

Charlop, M. H., & Trasowech, J. B. (1991). Increasing autistic children's daily spontaneous speech. *Journal of Applied Behavior Analysis, 24,* 247-261.

Charlop, M. H., & Walsh, M. (1986). Increasing autistic children's spontaneous verbalizations of affection through time delay and modeling. *Journal of Applied Behavior Analysis, 19,* 307-314.

Charlop, M. H., Kurtz, P. F., & Casey, F. G. (1990). Use of aberrant behaviors as reinforcers for autistic children. *Journal of Applied Behavior Analysis, 23,* 163-181.

Charlop, M. H., Kurtz, P. F., & Milstein, J. P. (1993). Too much reinforcement, too little behavior: Assessing different reinforcement schedules in conjunction with task variation with autistic children. *Journal of Applied Behavior Analysis, 26*, 225-239.

Charlop, M. H., Schreibman, L., & Thibodeau, M. G. (1985). Increasing spontaneous verbal responding in autistic children using a time delay procedure. *Journal of Applied Behavior Analysis, 18*, 155-166.

Charlop-Christy, M. H., & Haymes, L. (1996). Using obsessions as reinforcers with and without mild reductive procedures to decrease inappropriate behaviors of children with autism. *Journal of Autism and Developmental Disorders, 26*, 527-546.

Charlop-Christy, M. H., & Haymes, L. (in press). Using autistic children's obsessions as token reinforcers to increase task response. *Journal of Autism and Developmental Disorders.*

Charlop-Christy, M. H., & Kelso, S. E. (1997). *How to treat the child with autism: A guide to treatment at the Claremont Autism Center.* Claremont, CA: Claremont McKenna College.

DeLeon, I. G., & Iwata, B. A. (1996). Evaluation of a multiple-stimulus presentation format for assessing reinforcer preferences. *Journal of Applied Behavior Analysis, 29*, 519-533.

Dunlap, G., & Koegel, R. L. (1980). Motivating autistic children through stimulus variation. *Journal of Applied Behavior Analysis, 13*, 619-627.

Egel, A. L. (1981). Reinforcer variation: Implications for motivating developmentally disabled children. *Journal of Applied Behavior Analysis, 14*, 345-350.

Halle, J. (1984). Natural environment language assessment and intervention with severely impaired preschoolers. *Topics in Early Childhood Special Education, 4*, 36-56.

Halle, J. W., Baer, D. M., & Spradlin, J. E. (1981). Teachers generalized use of delay as a stimulus control procedure to increase language use in handicapped children. *Journal of Applied Behavior Analysis, 14*, 389-409.

Halle, J., Marshall, A.M., & Spradlin, J. E. (1979). Time delay: A technique to increase language use and facilitate generalization in retarded children. *Journal of Applied Behavior Analysis, 12*, 431-439.

Hart, B., & Risley, T. R. (1975). Incidental teaching of language in the preschool. *Journal of Applied Behavior Analysis, 8*, 411-420.

Iwata, B. A., Dorsey, M. F., Slifer, K. J., Bauman, K. E., & Richman, G. S. (1994). Toward a functional analysis of self-injury. *Journal of Applied Behavior Analysis, 27*, 197-209.

Kelso, S., & Charlop-Christy, M. H. (May 1996). *A study of age at intervention in an evaluation of a behavioral treatment program for children with autism: A preliminary report.* Poster session presented at the annual meeting of the Association for Behavior Analysis, San Francisco, CA.

Koegel, R. L., & Koegel, L. K. (1986). Promoting generalized treatment gains through direct instruction of self-monitoring procedures. *Direct Instruction News, 5,* 13-15.

Koegel, R. L., O'Dell, M. C., & Dunlap, G. (1988). Motivating speech use in nonverbal autistic children by reinforcing attempts. *Journal of Autism and Developmental Disorders, 18,* 525-537.

Koegel, R. L., O'Dell, M. C., & Koegel, L. K. (1987). A natural language paradigm for teaching non-verbal autistic children. *Journal of Autism and Developmental Disorders, 17,* 187-199.

Koegel, R. L., & Rincover, A. (1977). Research on the difference between generalization and maintenance in extra-therapy responding. *Journal of Applied Behavior Analysis, 10,* 1-12.

Koegel, R. L., Schreibman, L., Good, A., Cerniglia, L., Murphy, C., & Koegel, L. K. (1989). *How to teach pivotal behaviors to children with autism.* Santa Barbara, CA: University of California.

Laski, K. E., Charlop, M. H., & Schreibman, L. (1988). Training parents to use the Natural Language Paradigm to increase their autistic children's speech. *Journal of Applied Behavior Analysis, 21,* 391-400.

Lovaas, O. I. (1981). *Teaching developmentally disabled children: The me book.* Austin, Texas: Pro-Ed, Inc.

Lovaas, O. I., Koegel, R. L., Simmons, J. Q., & Stevens-Long, J. (1973) Some generalization and follow-up measures on autistic children in behavior therapy. *Journal of Applied Behavior Analysis, 6,* 131-166.

Michael, J. (1982). Distinguishing between the discriminative and motivational functions of stimuli. *Journal of the Experimental Analysis of Behavior, 37,* 149-155.

Michael, J. (1993). Establishing operations. *The Behavior Analyst, 16,* 191-206.

McGee, G. G., Krantz, P. J., & McClannahan, L. E. (1985). The facilitative effects of incidental teaching on preposition use by autistic children. *Journal of Applied Behavior Analysis, 18,* 17-31.

Nelson, K. (1973). Structure and strategy in learning to talk. *Monographs of the Society for Research in Child Development, 38* (No. 149).

Pierce, K., & Schreibman, L. (1995). Increasing complex social behaviors in children with autism via peer-implemented pivotal response training. *Journal of Applied Behavior Analysis, 28,* 285-295.

Rogers-Warren, A., & Warren, S. F. (1980). Facilitating the display of newly trained language in children. *Behavior Modification, 4,* 361-382.

Schreibman, L. (1988). *Autism.* Newbury Park, CA: Sage Publishing.

Schreibman, L., & Charlop-Christy M. H. (in press). Autism. In T. J. Ollendick & M. Hersen (Eds.), *Handbook of child psychopathology (2nd ed.).* New York, NY: Plenum.

Schreibman, L., Kaneko, W. M., & Koegel, R. L. (1991). Positive affect of parents of autistic children: A comparison across two teaching techniques. *Behavior Therapy, 22*, 479-490.

Schreibman, L., & Koegel, R. L. (in press). Training for parents of children with autism: Pivotal responses and generalization. In P. S. Jensen & E. D. Hibbs (Eds) *Psychosocial Treatment Research with Children and Adolescents*. Washington D. C.: American Psychological Association.

Stahmer, A. (1995). Teaching symbolic play skills to children with autism using Pivotal Response Training. *Journal of Autism and Developmental Disorders, 25*, 123-141.

Stokes, T. F., & Baer, D. M. (1977). An implicit technology of generalization. *Journal of Applied Behavior Analysis, 10*, 349-367.

Valdez, A. C. (1998). *Increasing play and speech behaviors in children with autism using play-speech therapy*. Unpublished senior thesis, Claremont McKenna College, Claremont, CA.

Discussion of Charlop-Christy and LeBlanc

Incorporating New Technology in the Treatment of Children With Autism

Thomas S. Higbee
University of Nevada

Charlop-Christy and LeBlanc successfully enumerate many of the challenges and obstacles faced by researchers and practitioners working with children diagnosed with autism. Traditional discrete trial teaching methods, while successful in teaching many verbal and nonverbal skills, certainly have limitations. Problems with generalization of skills to new settings, maintenance of acquired skills, and difficulties with spontaneity are sometimes encountered. Appropriate play and social behaviors can also be difficult to teach using discrete trial methods. The naturalistic teaching strategies described in this chapter appear to provide solutions to some of these problems.

The success of naturalistic teaching strategies is encouraging, but does not necessarily mean it is time to abandon discrete trial methods in favor of these alternative approaches. Discrete trial teaching has come a long way from the procedures outlined by Lovaas (1981) and cited by Charlop-Christy and LeBlanc. Programs such as the New England Center for Children, Princeton Child Development Institute, and the autism programs at the University of Nevada, just to name a few, are working to refine discrete trial methods by incorporating the results of current basic and applied research. Unfortunately, as is the case with much behavioral research in the area of early childhood autism, these procedural advances are not published and disseminated as often as they need to be.

Many skills can be taught rapidly and efficiently using current discrete trial methods. The utility of discrete trial teaching has been at least as well documented as that of naturalistic teaching methods. Luckily, the two approaches are not incompatible, so we are not forced to choose one or the other. Children with autism display many behavioral deficits and excesses that may respond better to one or the other teaching methods. A comprehensive treatment package capitalizing on the strengths of both naturalistic and discrete trial teaching strategies could be used to address the core deficits of autism. Many of the topics presented by Charlop-Christy and LeBlanc warrant further discussion. A few of these important issues are discussed below.

Enhancing Motivation

Charlop-Christy and LeBlanc detail the importance of child motivation in intervention practices. The authors briefly mention a relatively new systematic applied technology, stimulus preference assessment, that has received increasing attention in the research literature. Stimulus preference assessments have been shown to accurately identify reinforcing stimuli for adults with developmental disabilities (e.g., Fisher et al., 1992); children with developmental disabilities (Paclawskyj & Vollmer, 1995); and children with attention-deficit/hyperactivity disorder (Northup, Jones, Broussard, & Vollmer, 1995). The applicability of this technology to the treatment of children with autism is apparent. Carr, Nicolson, and Higbee (1998) recently developed a brief stimulus preference assessment designed specifically for children with autism. The assessment only takes about two minutes to administer and has been shown to produce results comparable to those achieved with lengthier methods. The short duration of the procedure enables those working with children with autism to assess potential reinforcers on a frequent basis. This is a necessary feature to match the ever-changing preferences often displayed by children with autism.

The research reported by Charlop-Christy and LeBlanc on the use of stereotypy, "obsessions," and other aberrant behaviors as reinforcers for appropriate behavior is interesting and warrants further exploration. As these behaviors typically occur at high rates in children with autism, it is likely that they could function as powerful reinforcers, as is suggested by the studies cited in this chapter (e.g., Charlop, Kurtz & Casey, 1990; Charlop-Christy & Haymes, 1996). Patel, Carr, and Dozier (1998) recently reported a case in which a stimulus preference assessment was used to identify stimuli associated and unassociated with stereotypy in a young girl diagnosed with autism. The authors found comparable reinforcement effects using both contingent stereotypy and empirically validated consequences. Future research is clearly needed to (a) further validate the use of stereotypy as a reinforcer, (b) assess the potential side effects of contingent stereotypy, and (c) incorporate stimulus preference assessments with contingent stereotypy methods. Whether discrete trial or naturalistic teaching strategies are used, the ability to predict reinforcers is a crucial component of intervention programs.

Family Involvement

Charlop-Christy and LeBlanc report both parental involvement and satisfaction with naturalistic teaching strategies (i.e., Natural Language Paradigm, Multiple Incidental Teaching Sessions). This is critical, as children with autism are likely to spend significantly more time with their parents and other family members than in traditional teaching settings. As suggested by the authors, traditional discrete trial procedures, which are often composed of mass training trials, may be too cumbersome to fit into parents' busy schedules. However, naturalistic teaching strategies, which are less structured and perhaps easier to learn, may more readily fit into parents' daily routines. The fact that parents are reported to enjoy using naturalistic teaching methods also suggests that they are likely to apply them. Using these techniques to provide learning opportunities in the natural home environment may lead to increased generalization of skills acquired in more formal teaching settings.

There is an unsettling lack of research on the use of siblings and age-peers in behavioral approaches to the treatment of children with autism. Only a few studies (e.g., McGee, Almeida, & Sulzer-Azaroff, 1992) have attempted to examine this practice. Because one of the ultimate goals of behavioral interventions for children with autism is to help the child acquire the necessary skills to be integrated into a regular education setting, it seems logical to establish siblings and age-peers as sources of reinforcement as early as possible. If a child spends most of the time with adults who are the main source of reinforcement, it should not be surprising when later attempts to increase the child's social behavior with respect to other children encounter difficulty. Perhaps future research will indicate the best way to incorporate siblings and age-appropriate peers into behavioral interventions for children with autism.

Programming for Generalization and Maintenance

A common criticism of traditional discrete trial methods, as discussed by Charlop-Christy and LeBlanc, is a lack of generalization and maintenance of acquired behaviors. The naturalistic teaching methods described in this chapter may help to ameliorate these problems. Providing learning opportunities in varied settings that more closely approximate the natural environment appears to facilitate generalization. The use of intermittent schedules of reinforcement during treatment has been shown to increase the durability of treatment gains. These and other strategies for generalization and maintenance are core features of naturalistic teaching methods that may need to be considered more carefully when discrete trial methods are employed.

Summary

The naturalistic teaching strategies outlined in this chapter target some of the core features of autism that have been more difficult to address with traditional discrete trial procedures. While an exclusive paradigm shift away from discrete trial methods may be premature, it is clear that children with autism could benefit by having naturalistic methods incorporated into their behavioral treatment programs. Being part of an evolving and progressive scientific approach, behavior-analytic programs for children with autism should be open to, and actively seek out, scientifically validated advances in treatment. Charlop-Christy and LeBlanc have done an excellent job summarizing such a direction.

References

Carr, J. E., Nicolson, A. C., & Higbee, T. S. (1998). *Evaluation of a brief method for assessing stimulus preference in children diagnosed with autism.* Manuscript submitted for publication.

Charlop, M. H., Kurtz, P. F., & Casey, F. G. (1992). Use of aberrant behaviors as reinforcers for autistic children. *Journal of Applied Behavior Analysis, 25,* 795-808.

Charlop-Christy, M. H., & Haymes, L. (1996). Using obsessions as reinforcers with and without mild reductive procedures to decrease inappropriate behaviors of children with autism. *Journal of Autism and Developmental Disorders, 26*, 527-546.

Fisher, W., Piazza, C. C., Bowman, L. G., Hagopian, L. P., Owens, J. C., & Slevin, I. (1992). A comparison of two approaches for identifying reinforcers for persons with severe and profound disabilities. *Journal of Applied Behavior Analysis, 25*, 491-498.

Lovaas, O. I. (1981). *Teaching developmentally disabled children: The me book.* Austin, TX: Pro-Ed.

Magee, G. G., Almeida, C. M., & Sulzer-Azaroff, B. (1992). Promoting reciprocal interactions via peer incidental teaching. *Journal of Applied Behavior Analysis, 25*, 117-126.

Northup, J., George, T., Jones, K., Broussard, C., & Vollmer, T. R. (1996). A comparison of reinforcer assessment methods: The utility of verbal and pictorial choice procedures. *Journal of Applied Behavior Analysis, 29*, 201-212.

Paclawskyj, T. R., & Vollmer, T. M. (1995). Reinforcer assessment for children with developmental disabilities and visual impairment. *Journal of Applied Behavior Analysis, 28*, 219-224.

Patel, M. R., Carr, J. E., & Dozier, C. L. (1998). *An evaluation of contingent access to stimuli associated with stereotypy in the acquisition of a non-vocal imitation response.* Manuscript submitted for publication.

Chapter 9

Peer-Mediated Intervention for Young Children With Autism: A 20-Year Retrospective[1]

Phillip S. Strain
University of Colorado at Denver
Frank Kohler
Allegheny-Singer Research Institute

The purpose of this paper is to provide the reader with an historical analysis of the development of our peer-mediated social skills intervention model from the mid-1970s to the present. We begin by tracking a series of precedent studies with adults as social skill intervention agents, and then proceed to present a developmental progression of peer-mediated studies.

Preliminary Studies with Adults as Intervention Agents

For 20 years now, we have been involved in research efforts aimed at remediating the social behavior deficits of young children with autism. This work has included a variety of intervention approaches, utilizing both adults and children as mediators of treatment. Our initial attempts at social behavior modification involved the exclusive use of teacher-manipulated antecedent and consequent events. By far the most dramatic changes in child behaviors were produced when we combined various antecedents (teachers' verbal and physical prompting) with contingent social attention from adults. In an initial study combining these tactics, a single preschool child was the primary target (Strain & Timm, 1974). The combined prompting and reinforcement strategy was equally effective when applied specifically to: a) the target child alone; or b) members of her peer group to encourage their social contact with her. Although the data system used in this study did not offer a separate account of individual peer group members' behavior, it appeared that intervention applied to the focal child had a parallel influence on several class members who were not direct recipients of intervention at a given moment.

In order more fully to portray this apparent "spillover" of treatment effect on non-target children, a second study in this sequence was initiated (Strain, Shores and Kerr, 1976). Here, we treated three preschool-age boys who varied considerably in their social behavior and overall skill development. The design allowed for a direct comparison of target subjects' behavior under these conditions: a) baseline, or no treatment; b) direct receipt of prompting and differential social reinforcement; and

c) member of a peer group not presently under intervention procedures. For two of the children, both direct and indirect treatment effects were obtained. That is, positive peer contacts increased when direct intervention tactics were applied, and when the two children observed the delivery of prompting and social reinforcement events to peers. For the third child, behavior change was noted only when intervention was applied directly.

Although we had been successful in making rather profound modifications in the social responsiveness of heretofore isolate, socially rejected children, it was abundantly clear that the children *immediately* returned to their isolate behavior patterns when intervention was terminated. In part, we suspected that the lack of maintenance was an artifact of the research designs employed. Specifically, when rich, relatively continuous reinforcement schedules are suddenly withdrawn, reinstated, withdrawn, and reinstated again, requirements for demonstrating experimental control usually are met. Ironically, when such powerful control of behavior is obtained, children may quickly discriminate that a particular time or setting is the occasion to be social, while all other occasions designate periods of isolation.

In an attempt to reduce the effects of sudden condition shifts on children's behavior, we later employed response-dependent fading of prompts and leaning of adult social reinforcement with two preschool boys with autism (Timm, Strain, & Eller, 1979). A third subject in this study was exposed to abrupt alterations between treatment (prompting and social reinforcement) and non-treatment conditions. After demonstrating experimental control over each subject's positive social behavior using a withdrawal of treatment design, two of the boys were placed under the response-dependent condition, the other under a response-independent condition. In the response-independent condition an *a priori* schedule of reducing the intensity of prompting and reinforcement resulted in a level of positive behavior identical to that produced when intervention was suddenly and completely withdrawn. However, when the other boys' level of positive interaction dictated how rapidly intervention was reduced, social behavior levels were identical to those produced during the most intensive prompting and reinforcement conditions. After a period of 40 days under the response-dependent conditions, the two boys positive interaction was being maintained by one prompting and one reinforcement event per five minutes.

It was at this rather optimistic point in the development of teacher-mediated intervention that our data became much less impressive. Going back to original observation protocols from our teacher-mediated treatment studies, we asked the question (via conditional probability analyses), "What are the immediate temporal consequences of reinforcement delivery." Simply put, we found that the immediate consequence of reinforcement delivery was a *termination* of child-child interaction. While the overall, day-to-day effect of treatment was an increase in the frequency of discrete social contacts, we feared that the intervention unintentionally limited the duration of social exchanges (Strain, 1980). The specific experimental analysis of this unintended treatment outcome was provided by Walker, Hops, and Greenwood (1981). Their study demonstrated that extended interaction episodes between children could only be developed when the reinforcement contingency was specifically applied to interactions of increased duration.

Given the treatment limitations and logistical complexities associated with adult-mediated intervention, we began a systematic study of the potential use of peers as instructional agents. From both naturalistic (e.g., Charlesworth & Hartup, 1967; Guralnick, 1981; Kohn, 1966) and intervention (e.g., Johnston & Johnston, 1981; Wahler, 1967) research it was clear that children exert a powerful influence on each other's social behavior. Sometimes this influence yields positive, maturing outcomes and sometimes it does not. If, indeed, peer influence plays a dominant role in the natural development of social and communicative competence, then it seems logical and reasonable to use peers in the purposeful development of children's social skills. Moreover, a fine-grain analysis of existing normative data on the social interactions of preschool children revealed that social exchanges were not begun by "prompt-like" statements from children, nor were they maintained by "praise-like" statements from interactants. Rather, our reading of the available developmental data indicated that interactions were begun and maintained by specific social overtures that were exchanged on an equitable, or reciprocal basis. Thus, our initial intervention effort was aimed at evaluating the functional effects of an increased level of social overtures or initiations on the social behavior of withdrawn children, who by definition rarely were exposed to any positive approach behaviors from peers.

Early Efficacy Studies of Peer-Mediated Interventions

In the first study of peer social initiations, six withdrawn preschool boys with autism were selected as target subjects (Strain, Shores & Timm, 1977). All children were enrolled in a developmentally integrated model program from which two typically developing boys were chosen as peer trainers. Four 20-min. training sessions were conducted with each of the typical peers. In these sessions the two boys learned and rehearsed a number of verbal and motoric behaviors to engage the target children in social play. First, the peers learned to initiate play by emitting phrases such as, "Come play," "Let's play ball." Next, the children were taught to engage in those motor behaviors that would naturally accompany specific verbal play overtures. For example, the peers would say "Let's play ball" and then roll a ball to the adult instructor. Each session contained 30 opportunities to practice appropriate initiations. On half of these occasions the experimenter would ignore the child's overtures for 10 seconds and then say, "Sometimes children will not want to play at first, but you need to keep asking them to play." Given the target subjects' usual response to play overtures, this "training to expect rejection" was considered to be an essential component of the instructional package. During an initial baseline period the target subjects rarely engaged in any positive interaction and their peers initiated only occasional social behaviors toward the six youngsters. When the peers were first instructed to play with the target subjects, two results were obtained. First, each target subject's responses to initiations immediately increased; and, second, the positive initiations of all but one child increased also. Treatment effects were replicated during subsequent return to baseline (low levels of initiations) and intervention phases. The one subject whose level of initiations did not increase was more severely language delayed than his peers. This child had a three word vocabulary, "Yes," "No," and "Mommy." However, he did not necessarily use these words on appropriate occasions.

In order to determine whether the effects produced by this peer-mediated intervention would generalize to another setting and maintain across a short time-span, we conducted a systematic replication in which three preschool-age boys were treated by one normally developing age-peer (Strain, 1977). The target children had IQ's of 55, 47, and 50 and ranged in age from 43 to 51 months-old. Two of the boys were echolalic and self-stimulatory. A peer training approach identical to that used by Strain et al. (1977) was employed with a 4 year-old boy. The intervention sessions in the withdrawal of treatment design took place in a small playroom. Generalization was assessed by observing the subjects in a regular free-play period in their classroom (the peer trainer was absent from this setting). Maintenance of behavior change across time was assessed by conducting generalization setting observations either immediately or 23 hours after intervention. Data from both intervention and generalization sessions showed an increase in social responding when intervention was in effect. For two of the subjects, a 5-fold increase in the frequency of positive social behavior occurred during treatment sessions. The remaining child's level of positive behavior improved only marginally. For the first two boys, an increase in positive social behavior was noted in the generalization sessions. Their positive contacts occurred at twice the level observed during baseline. The child who was affected minimally in the treatment setting showed no sign of generalized behavior change. Maintenance effects were noted also for the first two children, as no differences in performance were noted for generalization sessions that occurred immediately after treatment or 23 hours later.

The nonprogrammed generalization and short-term maintenance of effects with the social initiation strategy represented a dramatic and positive departure from our earlier adult-mediated treatment studies. What remained the same was the wide inter-subject variability in responsiveness to intervention. The child who showed little improvement had a lower baseline level of positive social behavior than his peers. However, clinical judgement suggested that other behavioral characteristics may have operated to diminish treatment effects with this child. This boy engaged in a high rate of self-stimulatory activity, and on occasion he would scream loudly when a peer interrupted his repetitive behavior. In a third experiment in this series, we attempted a more precise study of the interaction between children's inappropriate behaviors and the impact of peer social initiations (Kerr, Ragland & Strain, 1978). When compared with children treated in earlier studies on peer social initiations, the subjects in this investigation engaged in more active social withdrawal from peers and adults and more extensive forms of challenging behavior.

Each of the three target children had been diagnosed as autistic. The first child, Sally, was a 7 year old and had a measured IQ of 35. She was echolalic, frequently avoided eye contact, and engaged in lint-picking, object twirling, and scratching of herself. The second child, Darrin, was a 9-year-old boy who obtained a Vineland Social Maturity Scale score of 36 months. His speech was unintelligible and he continually engaged in some form of self-stimulation, including thumb sucking, twirling objects, finger-tapping, and tongue-clicking. The final subject, Dennis, was a 9 year-old boy who obtained an IQ score of 64. He had a history of petit mal seizures and bizarre verbalizations. At the time he participated in the peer-mediated treatment, Dennis' primary verbal behavior involved his fantasy of being a car. Also, Dennis was observed to bite and pinch himself when adults made requests of him. The peer trainer in this study was a 10 year-old boy who was enrolled in a class for children with learning and behavior problems. He had a long history of academic failure, disruptive classroom behavior, and verbal aggression toward adults. However, he was a child who got along quite well with his peers. The original peer training approach was modified slightly to accommodate the maladaptive behaviors exhibited by the target children. When the experimenter did not respond positively to initiations by the peer trainer she exhibited some of the self-stimulatory and avoidance behavior typical of the target subjects. The peer social initiation strategy produced an immediate increase in positive social behavior by each subject. In return to baseline and subsequent intervention conditions the treatment effect was replicated. Besides an increase in positive responding, the social initiation treatment had a tendency to increase negative interactions by Sally and Darrin, especially during the first several days of each intervention phase. The peer trainer often interrupted Sally and Darrin while they were engaged in some self-stimulatory activity. When this happened, these children would often scream and run away. After the first day that this situation occurred, the experimenter made sure to remind the peer after each session that sometimes children would respond this way.

A particularly significant outcome of the Ragland et al. (1978) study was the abrupt and substantial change in each subject's positive behavior. A number of our colleagues suggested that these low functioning target children could not, in fact, have been "truly autistic" and respond as they did to the social initiation procedure. Subsequently, we obtained three independent psychiatric evaluations of the three children in which each assessor used DSM-III diagnostic criteria. The psychiatrists were unanimous in their diagnosis of autism. Our explanation for the children's sudden behavior change is two-fold. First, the behavior patterns of children with autism is non-structured settings suggest to us a preference for stereotypic as opposed to social activity, not an active aversion for peer contact. Second, the isolate behavior of these children must be viewed, in part, as a function of the developmentally homogenous, socially unresponsive environments in which they are most often taught. We are not suggesting that developmentally segregated programming is an etiological variable in these children's withdrawn behavior, but it certainly serves to maintain socially unresponsive behavior.

Because of the controversy surrounding the application of the peer social initiation tactic with low functioning autistic children, a systematic replication was undertaken (Kerr, Ragland & Strain, 1979). We were also interested in seeing if negative behavior side-effects were limited to the social initiation procedures or a function of intervention in general. Four elementary-age children with autism served as target subjects. Earl was a 9 year-old boy who obtained an IQ score of 38. He had begun psychiatric treatment at age three because of his bizarre, stereotypic behavior. At the time of the study he was not toilet trained, he often cried for long periods of time, and was observed to engage in a high rate of stereotypic activity. Most of his verbal behavior was composed of repetitiously calling his own name. Sue was 10 year-old girl who was echolalic and extremely oppositional to adults' requests. She was also observed to tantrum when approached by peers. Tom was a 10 year-old boy who engaged in a high rate of stereotypic behavior and unintelligible verbalizations. He obtained an IQ score of 44. The final subject, Carl, was a 10 year-old boy who was described as hyperactive, and non-responsive to adults' requests. During a typical free-play period he would pull fabric from the carpet, slap a ball against the wall, and giggle. Carl was described by the school psychologist as "untestable."

One-half of the peer training was identical to that employed by Ragland et al. (1978). During the remaining portion, the peer was taught a prompting and reinforcement strategy. Here, the experimenter told the peer that he would be getting two of the children at a time to play with each other. The peer was instructed to rehearse such prompting statements as: "Roll the ball to _____," " "Give _____ a block," "Push the truck to _____." Later, the peers began to practice such praise statements as: "Good _____," "That's the way to play," "Very nice _____." The study employed two separate withdrawal of treatment designs (ABAC and ACAB), with two subjects exposed to each order of treatment. Sue and Carl composed one dyad for treatment while Tom and Earl were paired during intervention periods. During the first intervention phase, the prompting and reinforcement treatment was applied to Sue and Carl. The initial intervention for Tom and Earl was composed of peer social initiations. These treatments were later reversed for the two dyads. A generalization assessment was conducted each day 23 hours after intervention. We found that: a) both treatment procedures resulted in an immediate and substantial increase in the level of positive social behavior by each child; b) both procedures resulted in slight increases in subjects' negative interactions; c) a comparable level of positive and negative behavior change was associated with the two treatment procedures; and, d) no generalized behavior change was associated with either treatment procedure.

In several studies using the social initiation treatment we found a direct relationship between initial baseline performance and the immediate and generalized outcome of treatment (Strain, 1977; Strain et al., 1977). Withdrawn children who displayed lower baseline levels of positive social behavior were somewhat less responsive to treatment (although differences were slight) than youngsters with a relatively higher baseline performance. However, when the social initiation treatment was applied to children who engaged in a high level of stereotypic activity, no relationship was noted between subjects' initial baseline performance and immediate or generalized outcomes (e.g., Ragland et al., 1978; Strain et al., 1979). Our initial explanation for these divergent findings was that stereotypic behavior may compete with or mask an existing social repertoire.

In an attempt experimentally to test our notion regarding the role of stereotypic behavior in mediating social outcomes, we replicated the Ragland et al. (1978) study with three mentally retarded children who engaged in high rates of repetitive behaviors (Strain, 1980). Throughout the first four phases of the withdrawal of treatment design only treatment-setting change occurred. At this point, a token response cost for stereotypic behavior was instituted in the generalization setting. Each child entered the generalization setting with 10 tokens (beads worn around the neck). Each episode of stereotypic activity was consequated by removing one bead. At the end of the session the child traded each bead for one raisin. The token system quickly reduced each child's's level of stereotypic behavior; and, each of the youngsters began to engage in a low, stable level of positive interaction. The token program was later withdrawn and reinstated with predictable outcomes.

Component Effectiveness

Having demonstrated the overall efficacy of the peer-mediated strategy, we next began to examine the specific components that are responsible for the consistent impact of peer initiation procedures. In one study, Strain and Kohler (1995) investigated the impact of four different variables. Seven preschool staff rated 24 sociodramatic, manipulative, and gross motor activities for their likelihood of facilitating interaction from three children with autism. Nine different activities rated as high, moderate, and low were then incorporated into daily play activities involving a child with autism and two typically developing peers. Immediately prior to each session, teachers also predicted each focal child's likely responsiveness or sociability for the upcoming activity (1-5 point Likert Scale). Teachers were asked to base their prediction on the child's general performance and cooperation during activities that occurred during the preceding 1.5 hrs of the day rather than the type of play materials or selection of participating peers. Following an initial baseline, all children in the class participated in social skills training to learn shares, play organizers, assistance, and general comments. Teachers then implemented an individual contingency to reinforce children's use of these skills. All three focal children showed considerable variability in their day to day interaction with peers. Results indicated that the amount/percentage of peer overtures and degree of focal child reciprocity correlated highly with target children's levels of social interaction. In contrast, teachers' selection/ratings of play materials and predictions about sociability did not correlate with children's daily interaction levels during either the baseline or intervention phases. This study represented an important step in understanding the range of person- and environment-specific variables that may contribute to the variability in children's social skill performance.

In another investigation, Kohler, Strain and Shearer (1992) examined the form and function of social overtures that typical children directed toward three preschoolers with autism. All children received social skills training for play organizer suggestions, share offers and requests, assistance offers and requests, and general comments. Following training, children participated in daily six minute play sessions in groups of three, including one focal child and two peers. The social overtures that typical peers directed to their playmates with autism were analyzed in three different ways. First, we examined the percentage of occurrence for each individual behavior. Second, we examined the impact of each overture on the immediate responses of the individual children with autism. Finally, the impact of each behavior that led to a positive response on the subsequent duration of focal child-peer interaction was examined. Results indicated that the four peer behaviors had differential topographical and functional properties. Shares and play organizers occurred on an average of 5-6 times per session, while assists and general comments averaged less than 2 occurrences. Shares and play organizers also generated the highest percentage of positive responses from all three children with autism (averages of 73% and 86%, respectively). Conversely, assistance and general comments produced positive responses on only 60% of their occasions. Yet, the assists that did produce positive responses led to interactions averaging 33.4 seconds in duration, compared to only 15-16 seconds for shares and play organizers. The finding that peers' social overtures can have different and conflicting functions creates an important individualization challenge for early childhood teachers and practitioners. The decision of which specific initiations to teach depends on one's view of the focal child's existing repertoire, what divergent behavioral functions are desired, and in what order.

In summary, our research has examined the specific procedural components that are responsible for the overall effectiveness of peer initiation procedures. Our studies suggest that the amount and topography of peers' social overtures are among the more salient and important intervention variables. Along with focal children's social reciprocity, these two variables represent the essential index of quality and fidelity for peer-mediated procedures. Studies that continue to examine the effectiveness of individual procedural components will ensure the most robust and long-lasting improvements in children's social and communication skills.

Procedural Practicality or Feasibility

Our earlier peer-mediated interventions required close and continuous monitoring from a trained teacher, who provided ongoing suggestions, directions, feedback, and praise to enhance the frequency and quality of children's social exchanges and play (see Strain & Odom, 1986). An extensive body of research has documented the teacher's role in facilitating children's social interactions. For example, Curry-Sontag (1997) examined contextual factors that influence the sociability of preschool children with disabilities within integrated and segregated classrooms. A range of classroom variables were coded, including children's activity type, grouping arrangement, and the focus and quality of teacher behavior. Results indicated that teacher prompting was the only variable that correlated with children's social interaction with peers.

Despite its importance, however, prompting can become excessive and even preclude teachers' customary implementation of peer-mediated procedures (Kohler & Strain, 1990). In addition, high levels of teacher involvement can also interfere with the children's independent interactions as well as their ability to perform newly learned social and communication skills in novel settings or over time. Due to a range of pragmatic concerns, then, we have begun to address strategies that enable children to exhibit high quality interaction with reduced or minimal levels of adult prompting.

One viable strategy entails modifying the procedure for reinforcing children's social exchanges. Individual reinforcement contingencies enable each member of a group to experience individual consequences based solely upon their own performance. Conversely, interdependent group contingencies require that the consequences received by all group members are partially dependent on their own performance, and partially dependent on the performance of all other group members. Researchers have reported that children participating in group contingencies exhibit a variety of behaviors to influence or support one another's performance, such as spontaneous prompts and encouragement (Alexander, Corbitt, & Smigel, 1976), approval (Greenwood et al., 1977), assistance (Bailey, Deal &, Switzer, 1977), and tutoring (Axelrod & Paluska, 1975). In an extensive review, Greenwood and Hops (1981) concluded that corollary peer group support is a consistent and reliable outcome of group-oriented contingencies. If so, then peer encouragement, reminders, and related behaviors could replace teacher prompts, acting as a more naturalistic source of support for preschool children's social exchanges.

We have conducted several studies to examine the efficacy of group-oriented contingencies for facilitating children's social and supportive interactions. In a first investigation, Kohler et al., (1990) found that individual and group-oriented procedures produced equal increases in the social interactions between two preschoolers with autism and their peers. However, neither contingency generated consistent levels of supportive behaviors from typically developing peers involved in play sessions. Given this finding, children were taught to provide supportive prompts to their typical friends and playmates with autism (e.g., "Remember to share so that we can earn a happy face"). Following this brief training, children continued to exhibit high levels of social and supportive exchanges with very few teacher prompts during a second group contingency phase.

In a follow-up study, Kohler et al., (1995) once again found that an interdependent group contingency generated few supportive behaviors until children had received explicit training for these responses. Once trained, however, children exhibited an average of 5-10 supportive overtures per six-minute session during two subsequent group contingency phases with no teacher prompting. Data analyses indicated that peers directed an equal proportion of supportive prompts to their playmates with autism and typically developing youngsters. In addition, these prompts generated positive/compliant responses from their recipients on over 90% of occasions. Surprisingly, focal child-peer interactions occasioned by supportive prompts extended for over 20 sec in duration, compared to 13 seconds for interactions lacking peer support. Besides reducing children's dependence on adult prompts, then, group contingencies produced corollary forms of support that were associated with improvements in the duration of children's social interactions.

Self-monitoring represents another viable strategy for enhancing children's independent social exchanges with peers. In one investigation, Shearer et al., (1996) examined the effects of a self-monitoring procedure on the engagement and social interaction of three preschoolers with autism. Each child participated in daily play activities with one typical peer. Following an initial baseline, two different interventions were implemented in an alternating fashion. A first procedure required an adult to prompt the children to exchange social overtures and move beads to record children's social interactions. Each child also received a small post-session reward if they had completed a criterion number of exchanges. On alternating days, children moved their own beads while the adult provided fewer prompts and continued to present the post-session reward. The child monitoring procedure was then implemented without any adult prompts during a maintenance phase. Results indicated that the adult and child monitoring procedures were equally effective in maintaining children's social engagement and interaction during the alternating treatment phase. In addition, the child procedure maintained children's independent exchanges during the maintenance phase.

In a third study, Strain et al., (1994) utilized a self-monitoring intervention to increase the social interactions of three preschoolers with autism. Each child participated in five minute play activities within both a home (siblings) and school (peers) setting. Following an initial baseline, teachers and parents conducted an intervention involving adult prompting, edible reinforcement contingent on children's positive exchanges, and focal children's self-monitoring of their social behaviors. Results indicated that this package increased each focal child's interactions with their peers and siblings. Interestingly, the school and home procedures produced comparable effects on some dimensions of focal children's social performance, while other outcomes were affected differentially. Finally, adult prompts and reinforcement were successfully faded within both the home and school settings.

In summary, then, we have conducted a series of studies to address the feasibility or practicality of peer-mediated interventions. Although there are several important dimensions of practicality, our primary goal has been to reduce children's dependence on adult prompts. While it is probably unrealistic to expect that preschoolers with autism will exhibit high quality interaction with no adult support, our studies indicate that group-oriented contingencies and self-monitoring represent viable methods for increasing children's independence and potential generalization and maintenance.

Procedural Efficiency

Our initial peer-mediated procedures were very structured and prescribed with regard to teacher and child involvement. Typically developing peers received formal social skills training and prompts to direct high levels of social overtures to their playmates with autism. Similarly, teachers followed prescribed protocols to set-up play activities, conduct social skills training, and prompt/facilitate children's social exchanges during play activities. Despite its effectiveness, however, several concerns arose related to the efficiency of this procedure. For one, the high degree of structure restricted the range of classroom activities where peer-mediated procedures could be incorporated. Indeed, our early interventions were limited to socio-dramatic, manipulative, gross motor, and other activities that related directly to children's play. Second, the high degree of structure limited teachers' role in planning and contributing to the development of peer-mediated interventions. Given these issues, our research over the past several years has addressed two questions: (1) can teachers implement peer-based procedures in a spontaneous or nonprescribed fashion; and (2) what are the benefits of this method of implementation?

In an initial pilot study, Kohler, Strain, and Goldstein (1994) asked four pre-school teachers to identify naturally occurring opportunities to facilitate children's social interaction during 30 minute gross motor activities (dancing, climber, slide, tricycle, etc.). Teachers organized large group games or activities involving all 10-12 children in the classroom. Throughout the course of these activities, teachers looked for natural or "ideal" opportunities to facilitate peer interaction, such as holding hands, telling another child to jump, tossing your friend the ball, etc. In contrast to our earlier interventions, teachers employed methods that appeared natural or suited to children's ongoing actions, such as giving suggestions for new play roles/themes, adding materials to activities that matched children's interest, etc. The four teachers showed considerable variability in their overall success, as children's mean percent of interaction ranged from 15% to 45% across teachers. In addition, each teacher also showed a great deal of variability in their individual effectiveness, as children's daily interaction levels ranged from 5% to 65% or more. When interviewed after the study, all four teachers reported that they used the same basic strategies, which appeared to work on some days, but not on others. Teachers also felt that this approach generated natural or high quality forms of peer interaction, but was difficult to implement successfully on a consistent basis.

In a second investigation, Kohler et al., (in press) compared two methods to address preschool children's IEP objectives. Six teachers conducted their sessions during a variety of different classroom activities. In accordance with the tactics described by Bricker and Woods-Cripe (1992), teachers were asked to employ the following practices: (a) embed antecedents for children's IEP objectives into the context of ongoing play activities and areas; (b) utilize or follow children's ongoing actions and interests as the impetus for providing instruction; and (c) provide antecedents and consequences that are natural and logically suited to children's actions. Teachers provided all antecedents for addressing children's skills during an initial baseline phase. Conversely, both the teacher and peers (under the teacher's directions) provided antecedents in a second phase. Results indicated that the combined naturalistic and peer-mediated procedure produced high levels of social interaction from nine of ten children with autism. Interestingly, teachers also addressed more IEP skills with the combined method. The involvement of typically developing peers apparently provided teachers with a richer context for facilitating children's social interaction and related developmental skills.

In summary, our research indicates that naturalistic teaching provides a mechanism or context for enabling teachers to apply peer-mediated procedures in a spontaneous or non-prescribed fashion. Furthermore, the combination of naturalistic and peer-mediated tactics appear to be an efficient method for facilitating children's social interaction and related developmental skills. The next section describes our efforts to apply peer-mediated procedures on an expanded or program-wide basis.

Applying Peer-Mediated Procedures on Program-Wide or Expanded Basis

The second author of this chapter recently completed a five-year project examining expanded peer-mediated interventions for preschoolers with autism. The project was initially designed to address a series of questions related to procedural feasibility, efficiency, and effectiveness. One of our primary goals was to ensure that peer-mediated interventions were expanded in nature, or had the following characteristics: (a) are incorporated into the full range of preschool activities; (b) address a wide variety of different developmental skills; (c) involve a substantial number of children with autism, typically developing youngsters, and teachers; and (d) occur on a regular and consistent basis.

Table 1 illustrates nine different peer-mediated interventions that were developed throughout a one year period (1993-1994 school year) in our model program (LEAP) for typically developing children and peers with autism (Cordisco & Strain, 1993). As the table shows, peer-mediated interventions were developed for a wide range of different activities, including art, science and cooking, pet care, gross motor, etc. All nine procedures involved at least one child with autism, one or more typically developing peers, and a teacher. It is important to note that teachers provided varying amounts of supervision and direction in these activities. For example, the teacher actually participated in board games (e.g., took turns) with the children. Similarly, teachers maintained direct involvement in the science/cooking, pet care, classroom helper, and gross motor activities. Conversely, several procedures required less teacher involvement, such as art, snack set-up, table time, and sociodramatic play. In all cases, the teacher's role and direction was dictated by the nature of the specific activity, targeted skills, and needs of participating children. Table 1 also illustrates the developmental skills that were targeted with each intervention as well as the social exchanges involving children with autism and their typical peers. The nine procedures addressed a wide range of skills related to

Table 1. Description and Focus of Nine Peer-Mediated Interventions Developed Over a One-Year Time Period

Description of Activity Targeted	Developmental skills	Targeted Social Exchanges
Play **board games** in groups of 4-5 with close teacher supervision.	Follow directions; count; auditory discrimination; match letters, shapes, etc.	Take turns; model desired responses; request and provide assistance, share.
Complete **art activities** in groups of 3-5 with varying levels of teacher supervision.	Generate and answer How, Why, Where, and If questions; cutting, drawing, and other fine motor skills; follow directions.	Share; cooperate; request and provide assistance, exchange ideas and suggestions; model desired responses.
Complete **science and cooking** activities in groups of 3-5 with close teacher supervision.	Generate and answer questions; hands-on experimentation and observation; make predictions; follow directions.	Take turns; cooperate; request and provide assistance; exchange ideas and predictions; share; model responses.
Set up **snack tables** in groups of 2 with minimal teacher supervision.	Count; plan and estimate necessary materials; follow directions.	Cooperate; exchange ideas in planning; model desired responses.
Complete **pet care** activities in groups of 2 with close teacher direction (feed gerbil, clean cage, etc).	Follow directions; hands-on experimentation and observation.	Take turns; cooperate; request and provide assistance; share; exchange ideas and suggestions; model responses.

Table 1. (Continued)

Description of Activity	Targeted Developmental Skills	Targeted Social Exchanges
Complete **table time** activities in groups of 2-3 with minimal teacher supervision (in accordance with directions from tape).	Count, sort, or match objects; identify prepositional relationships, letters, or shapes; follow directions.	Take turns; cooperate; request and provide assistance; share; exchange suggestions; model desired responses.
Complete **classroom helper** activities in groups of 2 with close teacher supervision (check weather, ring bell for transition).	Follow directions; count; identify letters and shapes; other pre-academic skills.	Take turns; cooperate; request and provide assistance; exchange ideas and suggestions; model desired responses.
Play in **socio-dramatic** activities in groups of 3-5 with moderate teacher supervision.	Experiential adaptation and simulation; appropriate thematic roles and actions.	Cooperate; share materials; exchange ideas and suggestions.
Engage in **gross motor** activities in groups of 10-12 with close teacher supervision.	Follow directions; range of movement; dancing and related gross motor skills.	Cooperate; take turns; model desired responses.

children's language, cognitive, social, and fine/gross motor domains. In addition, focal children and peers fulfilled a wide range of social exchanges, including taking turns, cooperating, modeling desired responses, sharing ideas and suggestions, etc.

Table 2 illustrates the number of participating classrooms, children with autism, typical peers, and teachers for each of these nine interventions. The LEAP program included a total of three preschool classes. Most peer-mediated procedures were implemented in 1 or 2 of these classes while the gross motor intervention occurred in all 3 rooms. Each individual classroom included a total of 12-13 children, including 3 youngsters with autism and 9-10 typically developing peers. As shown in Table 2, the peer-mediated procedures involved varying numbers of focal and typically developing participants. Finally, a range of 1-4 teachers implemented these interventions.

Table 3 illustrates the implementation schedule for each peer-mediated procedure. As the table shows, the activities ranged from 5-15 minutes in duration and occurred from two to eight times per week in each class. Procedures that involved more than two focal children (in the same class) sometimes occurred more than 4-5 times a week, as teachers may have repeated the activity for different children. The procedures also occurred for varying lengths of time, ranging from 4 weeks for the gross and sociodramatic play to 19 weeks for board games. Based on the duration and frequency of implementation, then, the activities resulted in a varying number of total intervention minutes for their recipients. It is important to note that all nine procedures did not occur at the same time, but were implemented over a 12 month period in a staggered fashion. The next section of this paper illustrates a case study for one child who received these expanded peer-mediated interventions over the one year time period.

Case Study for One Individual Child With Autism

The purpose of this final section is to illustrate a case study of one preschool boy who participated in this project. This child was 2 yrs, 11 mos when he enrolled in the preschool program. At this time, he had a diagnosis of moderately autistic on the Childhood Autism Rating Scale and scored at or below the 25th percentile on all categories of the McCarthy's Scale of Children's Abilities. The child was 6 yrs, 4 months when he left the LEAP program, having spent a total of 3 yrs, 5 months in the preschool.

Table 4 illustrates the peer-mediated interventions that this boy participated in during the one year period corresponding with Table 1. Like all children with autism enrolled in the program, this child participated in a variety of peer-mediated interventions that were suited to his unique developmental needs and abilities.

A first and primary objective of peer-mediated interventions is to alter the context for children's participation in routine preschool activities. Indeed, our assessments indicate that children with autism and typically developing youngsters both exhibit high levels of appropriate engagement in typical classroom situations.

Table 2. Number of Classrooms, Children, and Teachers Participating in Nine Different Peer-Mediated Interventions

Procedure	Number of classes implementing procedure (3 total)	Ratio of participating to total focal children	Ratio of participating to total peers	Ratio of participating to total teachers
Board Games	2	2/6	7/20	3/4
Art	1	2/3	6/10	2/2
Science and Cooking	1	2/3	6/10	1/2
Set up snack table	1	2/3	10/10	2/2
Pet care	1	3/3	9/10	1/2
Table time	2	3/6	6/19	3/4
Classroom helper	1	3/3	5/10	2/2
Sociodramatic play	2	3/6	9/19	2/4
Gross motor play	3	7/9	9/29	4/6

Table 3

Average Implementation Time (per participating classroom) for Nine Different Peer-Mediated Interventions

Peer-Mediated Procedure	Activity length	Weekly occurrences	Total weeks	Total sessions	Total time of implementation
Board Games	15 min	3	19	57	14 hrs
Art	10 min	3	6	18	3 hrs
Science and Cooking	10 min	2	5	10	1.5 hrs
Set up snack table	5 min	4	10	40	3 hrs
Pet care	12 min	2	7	14	2.5 hrs
Table time	15 min	6	14	84	21 hrs
Classroom helper	5 min	3	11	33	2.5 hrs
Sociodramatic play	10 min	6	4	24	4 hrs
Gross motor play	10 min	8	4	32	5 hrs

That is, both groups climb on gross motor equipment, manipulate blocks and other toys, and engage in other activity related actions. The primary difference between these groups lies in the context for their participation. Without formal intervention, preschoolers with autism exhibit nearly all of their engagement in a solitary fashion or in the context of teacher interactions (usually initiated by the teacher). Conversely, typically developing youngsters exhibit 20-30% of their participation in the context of peer interactions.

Table 5 illustrates the boy's performance during two separate observational rounds that were conducted during the 1993-1994 school year. Both observations extended for 30 min and occurred during an activity where one or more peer-mediated interventions were embedded. It is important to note that interventions did not occur during the entire observational period, but only for some portion of the total 30 min observation period. In any case, Table 5 shows that the child's active engagement was 59% and 73% during these two observation periods. More significant is the fact that 31% to 42% of this child's participation occurred within the context of peer interaction (i.e., verbal or nonverbal exchanges, associative play, etc.). Upon program entry, this child showed **no** peer interactions. Given the low levels of social engagement typically observed from children with autism, these data indicate that the peer-mediated strategies were effective in increasing this child's social participation to a level equal or superior to that found with typically developing peers. It is important to note that this child also entered a regular education kindergarten after leaving the preschool program, and has participated successfully in regular education classes during his first and second grade years.

Table 4. Peer-Mediated Interventions Received by One Preschool Child With Autism Over a One-Year Time Period

Procedure	Dates of Implementation	Total number of sessions received	Total minutes of intervention
Art	12/15/93 - 02/12/94	6	60
Science and Cooking	9/30/93 - 12/12/94	5	50
Table time	02/03/94 - 5/30/94	14	210
Classroom helper	12/03/93 - 4/30/94	8	40
Socio-dramatic play	06/15/93 - 08/04/93	17	170
Total		49	530 (5.5 hrs)

Conclusions

The peer-mediated strategies used to influence the development of social skills among young children with autism have lead us to the following, tentative conclusions. Conclusion One: Young children with autism may not need skill training as we know it to achieve good social outcomes. Our initial conceptualization of the social, or shall we say, non-social repertoire of these children was based on a clear behavioral deficit model. Accordingly, we began by having adults dutifully prompt and reinforce ever more sophisticated social responses between age peers. Frankly, the whole notion of peer-mediated intervention was born out of this treatment and conceptual dead-end. Not only did we shift intervention paradigms, but we also

Table 5. Case Study of One Child's Performance During 30 Min Activities Where Peer-Mediated Interventions Were Embedded

Observational Round	Date	Percentage of active engagement	Percentage of engagement involving peers
1	September, 1993	59%	31%
2	April, 1994	73%	42%

shifted our most basic conceptualization of these children's social repertoire. Specifically, we entertained the possibility of a performance deficit model in which isolate behavior is maintained by ecologies that yield few, if any, peer social encounters, and in which active avoidance behaviors punish peer approaches.

Today, we know that over 80 young children with autism have demonstrated the following behavior changes, without specific adult instruction: a) increased their time spent in positive peer interaction; b) increased the length of their social encounters; c) approximated reciprocity in their social exchanges after two years in daily intervention; d) generalized social behaviors to new settings and peers after two years in daily intervention; and e) increased specific behaviors we know lead to friendship formation, including sharing, organizing play, helping others, and showing affection.

These behavior changes are all under the functional control of increased levels of persistent social overtures from age-peers. How is this possible? We invite the consideration of four possibilities, all of which have some empirical backing with varying numbers of clients.

First, the intervention coincidentally is an extinction paradigm for socially avoidant behavior, which has masked a more accomplished repertoire. Probably the best evidence we have for this explanation is a 3 to 5 day extinction burst for negative interactions during initial social initiation phases coupled with day one, positive intervention effects for *all* subjects. Second, the fact that we occasionally see novel behaviors and chains of behaviors by clients leads us to believe that peer imitation is operating. Third, most studies have had multiple intervention agents, using a "loose training paradigm" comprised of many and varied initiations. Perhaps the generalization we see is attributable to this haphazard use of generalization programming. Fourth, peers know what they like, in the social sense, and work till they get encounters that are satisfying to them. That is, their aim is not simply to beat baseline, but to engage in enjoyable social encounters. We have come to believe that it is essential to have the ultimate social validity agents as interventionists for children's socially isolate behavior.

Conclusion Two: Primarily being around other people with limited social repertoires is deleterious to social development. From a rather extensive series of studies we know the following about developmentally segregated contexts for preschoolers with autism: 1) They can occur in any administrative arrangement. That is, children can become isolated and skills extinguished in sloppy integrated administrative settings. 2) Lack of familiarity breeds contempt on the part of typical peers. That is, young typical children often develop negative stereotypes about age-peers with disabilities. This stereotyping is ameliorated by their participation as intervention agents. 3) Newly acquired social behaviors are readily extinguished in developmentally segregated settings. 4) When around other children with autism, these youngsters engage in more autistic-like behaviors, increasing the likelihood of peer rejection and reducing the likelihood of socially appropriate behaviors occurring. 5) Once you start school in a developmentally segregated setting there is a 90% probability that you will always be there. It is the equivalent of life without parole. These data have been misused often to advocate for cost-driven, mean-spirited, or just plain ill-advised attempts at inclusive education. A more careful reading of the studies will hopefully lead to the conclusion that we never saw inclusion as an outcome, merely a context to best treat social deficits and ensure treatment gains across settings and time. In fact, the baseline phase in many of our studies directly show the developmentally trivial results produced by a placement as outcome mentality.

Conclusion Three: Excellent treatment fidelity can overcome zero baselines, high levels of stereotypies, and negative social history among peers. We have spent considerable effort aimed at answering the question, "For whom does this tactic work best?" We followed the usual suspects: a) IQ, b) age, c) interfering repertoire, and the like. The good news is that we cannot predict outcome based on child characteristics; the bad news is that there are generous and not-so-generous interpretations of this fact. On the one hand, we might have a really powerful intervention paradigm. On the other, maybe we have massive measurement error, particularly in regard to psychometric-based indices of intervention co-variates. Or perhaps we are too myopic to see the logical predictors. Or, given the heterogeneity of autism, maybe 80 subjects are not sufficient to study client/intervention interactions. What we know for certain about the client/intervention interaction equation is that treatment fidelity corresponds with outcome at an extraordinarily high level and, if children engage in heightened stereotypies when they are approached, it is best to install some contemporaneous behavior reduction program to optimize the peer-mediated outcomes.

Conclusion Four: Typical peers receive multiple benefits from their intervention involvement and no negative consequences. When compared to children nominated as preschool "stars" by their teachers, children who have engaged in intervention for one year are: a) less likely to engage in inappropriate behaviors; b) experiencing the same rate of intellectual and communicative development; c) more social with other typical kids; d) judged to be more socially competent by teachers; and e) less likely to have developed negative stereotypes about disability in the preschool years, as discussed earlier.

References

Alexander, R. N., Corbitt, T. F., & Smigel, J. (1976). The effects of individual and group consequences on school attendance and curfew violations with predelinquent adolescents. *Journal of Applied Behavior Analysis, 9,* 221-226.

Axelrod, S., & Paluska, J. (1975). A component analysis of the effects of a classroom spelling program. In E. Ramp & G. Semb (Eds.), *Behavior analysis: Areas of research and application* (pp. 277-282). Englewood Cliffs, NJ: Prentice-Hall.

Bricker, D., & Woods-Cripe, J. J. (1992). *An activity-based approach to early intervention.* Baltimore: Paul H. Brookes.

Charlesworth, R., & Hartup W. W. (1967). Positive social reinforcement in the nursery school peer group. *Child Development, 38,* 993-1002.

Curry-Sontag, J. (1997). Contextual factors influencing the sociability of preschool children with disabilities in integrated and segregated classrooms. *Exceptional Children, 63,* 389-404.

Greenwood, C.R., & Hops, H. (1981). Group-oriented contingencies and peer behavior change. In P.S. Strain (Ed.), *The utilization of classroom peers as behavior change agents* (pp. 189-255). New York: Plenum.

Greenwood, C. R., Walker, H. M., & Hops, H. (1977). Some issues in social interaction/withdrawal assessment. *Exceptional Children, 43,* 490-499.

Guralnick, M. J. (1981). Peer influences on the development of communicative competence. In P. S. Strain (Ed.), *The utilization of classroom peers as behavior change agents.* New York: Plenum.

Kohler, F. W., and Strain, P. S. (1990). Peer-Assisted Interventions: Early promises, notable achievements and future aspirations. *Clinical Psychology Review, 22,* 441-452.

Kohler, F. W., Strain, P. S., & Goldstein, H. (1994). Examining teachers' use of naturalistic strategies to facilitate interactions between preschoolers with autism and their peers. Allegheny Singer Research Institute, Pittsburgh, PA.

Kohler, F. W., Strain, P. S., Hoyson, M., Davis, L., Donina, W. M., & Rapp, N. (1995). Using a group-oriented contingency to increase social interactions between children with autism and their peers: A preliminary analysis of corollary supportive behaviors. *Behavior Modification, 19,* 10-32.

Kohler, F. W., Strain, P. S., Hoyson, M., & Jamieson, B. (In press). Merging naturalistic and peer-based strategies to address the IEP objectives of preschoolers with autism: An examination of structural and child behavior outcomes. *Focus on Autism and Other Developmental Disabilities.*

Kohler, F. W., Strain, P. S., Maretsky, S., & DeCesare, L. (1990). Promoting positive and supportive interactions between preschoolers: An analysis of group-oriented contingencies. *Journal of Early Intervention, 14,* 327-341.

Kohler, F. W., Strain, P. S., & Shearer, D. D. (1992). The overtures of preschool social skill intervention agents: Differential rates, forms, and functions. *Behavior Modification, 16,* 525-542.

Kohn, M. (1966). The child as a determinant of his peers' approach to him. *Journal of Genetic Psychology, 109,* 91-100.

Johnston, D. W., & Johnston, R. T. (1981). Effects of cooperative and individualistic learning contingencies on interethnic interaction. *Journal of Educational Psychology, 73,* 444-449.

Ragland, E. U., Kerr, M. M., & Strain, P. S. (1978). Effects of peer social initiations on the behavior of withdrawn autistic children. *Behavior Modification, 2,* 565-578.

Shearer, D. D., Kohler, F. W., Buchan, K. A., & McCullough, K. M. (1996). Promoting independent interactions between preschoolers with autism and their nondisabled peers: An analysis of self-monitoring. *Early Education and Development, 7,* 205-220.

Strain, P. S. (1977). Training and generalization effects of peer social initiations on withdrawn preschool children. *Journal of Abnormal Child Psychology, 5,* 445-455.

Strain, P. S. (1980). Social behavior programming with severely emotionally disturbed and autistic children. In B. Wilcox & A. Thompson (Eds.), *Critical issues in educating autistic children and youth.* Washington, D. C.: Bureau of Education for the Handicapped.

Strain, P. S., & Cordisco, L. (1993). The LEAP preschool model: Description and outcomes. In S. Harris & J. Handleman (Eds.), *Preschool education programs for children with autism.* Austin: Pro-ed.

Strain, P. S., Kerr, M. M., & Ragland, E. U. (1979). Effects of peer-mediated social initiations and prompting/reinforcement procedures on the social behavior of autistic children. *Journal of Autism and Developmental Disorders, 9,* 41-54.

Strain, P. S., & Kohler, F. W. (1995). Analyzing predictors of daily social skill performance. *Behavioral Disorders, 21,* 79-88.

Strain, P. S., Kohler, F. W., Storey, K., & Danko, C. D. (1994). Teaching preschoolers with autism to self-monitor their social interactions: An analysis of results in home and school settings. *Journal of Emotional and Behavioral Disorders, 2,* 78-88.

Strain, P. S., & Odom, S. L. (1986). Peer social initiations: Effective interventions for social skills development of exceptional children. *Exceptional Children, 52,* 543-551.

Strain, P. S., Shores, R. E., & Kerr, M. M. (1976). An experimental analysis of "spillover" effects on social interaction among behaviorally handicapped preschool children. *Journal of Applied Behavior Analysis, 9,* 31-40.

Strain, P. S., Shores, R. E., & Timm, M. A. (1977). Effects of peer initiations on the social behavior of withdrawn preschoolers. *Journal of Applied Behavior Analysis, 10,* 289-298.

Strain, P. S., & Timm, M. A. (1974). An experimental analysis of social interaction between a behaviorally disordered preschool child and her classroom peers. *Journal of Applied Behavior Analysis, 7,* 583-590.

Switzer, E. B., Deal, T. E., & Bailey, J. S. (1977). The reduction of stealing in second graders using a group-contingency. *Journal of Applied Behavior Analysis, 10,* 267-272.

Timm, M. A., Strain, P. S., & Eller, P. H. (1979). Effects of systematic, response-dependent fading and thinning procedures on the maintenance of child-child interaction. *Journal of Applied Behavior Analysis, 12,* 308.

Wahler, R. G. (1967). Child-child interactions in free field settings: Some experimental analyses. *Journal of Experimental Child Psychology, 5,* 278-293.

Walker, H. M., Hops, H., & Greenwood, C. R. (1981). RECESS: Research and development of a behavior management package for remediating social aggression in the school setting. In P. S. Strain (Ed.), *The utilization of classroom peers as behavior change agents* (pp. 261-303). New York & London: Plenum.

1. The context of this chapter is based, in part, on a paper by the authors published in *Seminars in Speech and Language Disorders*, 1998.

Discussion of Strain and Kohler

Toward a Definition of Social Behavior

Patrick M. Ghezzi
University of Nevada

Judging by the voluminous literature on the topic, the development and remediation of social behavior in young children is regarded as an important area for study. The strong interest is especially evident over the last two decades, a period marked initially by an outpouring of behavior-analytic research, and later by the establishment of numerous empirically based clinical interventions and classroom applications.

In tracing the development of his own work over roughly the same period, Dr. Strain does much more than give us a retrospective appreciation of his seminal contributions to understanding and remediating child social behavior. Specifically, he exposes a path to solving a thorny conceptual issue that has plagued the field for many years, namely, how to define social behavior in a manner that aligns theory, research, and practice.

The aim of this commentary is three-fold: (a) to identify a few problems that stem from an improvident regard for a conceptual definition of child social behavior; (b) to highlight B. F. Skinner's and J. R. Kantor's perspectives on social behavior, with an eye toward uncovering in the writings of these two architects of contemporary behavior theory a coherent conceptual approach to social behavior; and, (c) to illustrate how the research and practice of Strain and his colleagues sheds some much-needed light on the problems at hand.

The Difficulty of Defining Social Behavior

Contained in virtually every research review and conceptual paper published over the past 20 years on the social behavior of young children is an initial discussion of how difficult it is to define the behavior(s) of interest. The sentiment expressed in the literature is that, like beauty and art, it is difficult to say precisely what social behavior is, yet we all seem to know it when we see it, and especially when we do not see it. Concluding that advances in the field will depend upon arriving at a coherent conceptual definition of social behavior, the reviews and papers blithely go on to document the progress that researchers have made in understanding how social behavior develops, how it has been measured, assessed, and evaluated, and how it can be remediated or taught in children who show delays or deficits in it.

Workers in the field obviously have been undeterred by the absence of a definition of social behavior that goes beyond the operations employed for its investigation. They have instead proceeded at full speed under the apparent influence of Skinner's (1972) position on defining psychological terms: "The ultimate criterion for the goodness of a concept [is] whether the scientist who uses the concept can operate successfully upon his material" (p. 383).

In view of the success that researchers have had in "operating upon" their material, the matter of pursuing a conceptual definition of child social behavior has the look of a red herring. On the other hand, success in behavior-analytic research is always a matter of degree, subject to considerations beyond the requisite demonstration of a functional relationship between a given class of behavior and an intervention designed to alter its occurrence (Baer, Wolf, & Risely, 1987).

One such consideration is the production of enduring, generalized behavior change. Unfortunetly, this has been very difficult to achieve in young children who have undergone social behavior training (Chandler, Lubeck, & Fowler, 1992). Indeed, poorly generalized and weakly maintained behavior is the norm, the main effect being to limit the utility of most training procedures to particular settings and arrangements of experimental conditions.

Outcomes of that sort can have a chilling affect on a field. Indeed, the apparent decline in recent years in interest in child social behavior may be a reflection of repeated failures to achieve enduring, generalized behavior change. In the face of those failures, many workers may have simply abandoned the field for greener pastures. Others with a higher tolerance for failure seem to have shifted the focus of their research away from simply demonstrating a treatment effect to questions that center on how generalized and maintained behavior change can be achieved (Chandler, et al., 1992). The work of Strain and his colleagues is a meaningful example of this, and, as we shall see in a moment, the success of their efforts may relate to a conceptual orientation that takes advantage of Skinner's and Kantor's views on social behavior.

Behavior Analysis of Social Behavior

Skinner (1953) defined social behavior as "the behavior of two or more people with respect to one another *or* in concert with a common environment" (p. 297, italics added). There are two things to note about this definition. First, in order for behavior to be called social, there evidently must be two people involved. Second, the first clause alludes to a class of social behavior that presumably is different from the class that is mentioned in the second clause. Respecting the distinction, events in the first clause may be termed "interpersonal." Events in the second clause have been identified, at one extreme, as cooperative, and at the other, competitive (Hake & Olvera, 1978).

Cooperative, Competitive, and Interpersonal Behavior

On Skinner's terms, a cooperative contingency is one "in which the reinforcement of two or more individuals depends upon the behavior of both or all of them"

(1953, p. 311). A clear example of the contingency is two men pulling on a rope that neither could pull alone. A competitive contingency, in contrast, is one in which "the behavior of one [individual] can be reinforced only at the cost of the reinforcement of the other [individual]" (1953, p. 311). Examples of competitive contingencies abound, yet what might be overlooked is that social behavior is not necessarily involved. For example, the child who takes the last toy from the toybox, leaving no toy for another child, has "cost" that other child, but the situation would be social only if it were shown that the behavior of taking the last toy was reinforced by its (presumably aversive) affect on the other child. If only the toy was the reinforcer, there would be no reason to distinguish the child's behavior as social. The point here is that while competitive behavior is not always social, cooperative behavior always is, by virtue of the requirement that reinforcement for one (or more) individual be dependent upon the behavior of at least one other individual.

While social behavior is sometimes cooperative and at other times competitive, much of the time it is neither, but is instead interpersonal. In this case, there are, after Skinner, simply "two or more people [behaving] with respect to one another" (1953, p. 297). There are no distinctive contingencies which call for a more or less equitable distribution of responses and/or reinforcers, as in cooperation, nor are there drastic deviations from equity, as in competition (Hake & Vukelich, 1978). Rather, what one individual does and says evokes behavior from a second individual, who in turn affects the first individual, and so forth, throughout the exchange. Skinner (1953) offered as the definitive example of interpersonal behavior a face-to-face conversation between two people. He depicted that situation as an "interlocking social system" characterized by "reciprocal interchange" and bound by "mutual reinforcement."

Explicit in Skinner's analysis of verbal behavior (1957) is that the social system with which an individual is interlocked is a language community wherein reciprocal interchanges occur between individual speakers and listeners who behave with respect to one another by means of conjoined vocal-verbal and gestural responses. Mutual reinforcement combines with other variables to establish and sustain interpersonal interactions. How speakers and listeners are able to respond to each other is, according to Skinner, a matter of learning the verbal practices of the group of which they are members.

There, then, is a brief account of Skinner's perspective on social behavior. Circumstances which give rise to cooperative and competitive interactions are distinguished from those that stimulate interpersonal interactions. These circumstances obviously are intermingled in ordinary life such that it may be practically impossible to disentangle one from the other. Under extraordinary circumstances, however, one may observe a child, for example, who displays excessive competitive behavior or deficient cooperative behavior, or who likewise shows excesses or deficits in the interpersonal domain. Our view is that the problem oftentimes is in the interpersonal domain. It follows from this that interventions aimed at remediating or teaching verbal-vocal and gestural behavior will have the greatest impact on the social life of a child.

Interbehavioral Analysis of Interpersonal Behavior

It is important to point out from the start that Kantor eschewed the term "social behavior," preferring instead to distinguish between "cultural behavior" and "interpersonal behavior." Kantor (1982) reserved the former term to identify the behaviors that a given individual performs in common with other members of a particular group, and used the latter term to describe everyday circumstances wherein individuals have "mutual influences upon each other" (1926, p. 290). He portrayed that situation as an "interplay of action" that ordinarily takes place between persons who are both "responding and highly responsive to" one another in a "momentary and spontaneous" fashion that he likened to "the infinite changes in the play of kaleidoscopic color" (1926, p. 291).

Kantor (1926) identified four types of interpersonal behavior. In one type, which he termed *autogenic*, an individual's behavior is "directed toward and remotely stimulated by various objects and persons which possess their particular stimulational functions because of the reacting individual's own interpretation and evaluation of those objects and persons" (1926, p. 296). Perhaps the most striking feature of the autogenic type of interpersonal behavior is that it is often evoked by inanimate objects. A familiar example of this is seen in young children who play and talk with dolls or stuffed animals as though those objects were alive. Another example is prayer and other acts of reverence that a person directs toward a religious deity (e.g., Christ) or toward a symbol for a deity (e.g., a crucifix). What these examples point out is that not all interpersonal behavior occurs in the explicit presence of other persons, but may instead occur with respect to things that have acquired the functions associated with other people.

A second type of interpersonal behavior is termed *homogenic*. "The central mark of distinction of this type," wrote Kantor, "is the fact that the primary interactions are with the reacting person himself" (Kantor, 1926, p. 298). Within this type, which Kantor also dubbed "self-stimulational," are private or covert behaviors, the most common of which is "having a conversation with yourself." Because other persons do not explicitly participate in this type of interaction, it joins the autogenic type as an example of interpersonal behavior that occurs in the absence of other persons.

A third type of interpersonal behavior, *heterogenic*, is illustrated by the "planning and plottings which individuals perform as direct responses to the activities of other individuals in whom they are interested or with whom they compete" (Kantor, 1926, p. 300). What is most distinctive about this type is that, whereas one person is stimulated by another person to behave in some manner, that other person is not immediately, or perhaps ever affected by, the person whose behavior he or she has stimulated. Kantor offered the example of the scholar who spends hours "scrutinizing, criticizing, and marshalling objections to the work of another scholar of a very different type of school of thought" (1926, p. 300). A related example is the young child who has been sent to her room for misbehaving, and while alone there rails aloud against her mother for the unjust manner in which she has been treated. (My youngest daughter used to do this, and now silently registers her complaints in a diary.) The explicit participation of another person is not necessary to evoke heterogenic behavior, thus in this respect it is similar to the autogenic and homogenic types of interpersonal behavior.

A fourth type of interpersonal behavior, *reciprogenic*, comes closest to conventional perspectives – Skinner's included – on social behavior. Kantor (1926) characterized reciprogenic behavior as a "very definite mutuality of interstimulation and interresponse" between two individuals who both are "aware of themselves as the source of stimulation for the other individual and as responding to the stimulational changes resulting in each other" (p. 310). Kantor assumed that "reciprogenic interpersonal situations are founded upon linguistic behavior" (1926, p. 306), and offered as the definitive example an ordinary, everyday conversation between two people.

Kantor (1977) eventually identified reciprogenic behavior as "referential linguistic behavior." He characterized referential behavior as bi-stimulational, meaning that a speaker, in making a linguistic response, is behaving with respect to two stimuli, the thing or event referred to (the "referent") and the listener. The listener, in turn, is also responding to two stimuli, the referent and the speaker. For Kantor, the moment-to-moment verbal-vocal and gestural interactions that unfold between speakers and listeners is the most typical of all human conduct.

There, then, is a brief account of Kantor's perspective on interpersonal behavior. Perhaps the most striking feature of his analysis is that of the four types he identified, three – autogenic, homogenic, and heterogenic – occur in the absence of other persons. In this regard, Kantor differs from conventional views which hold that at least two people must be interacting with one another in order for their individual or collective behavior to be identified as social (for an extended discussion on this point, see Parrott, 1983). We should not be surprised, however, to find that (a) inanimate objects can exert stimulus control over behavior that is ordinarily controlled by other persons, (b) one's behavior can simulate acts which are indistinguishable from those which are stimulated by other persons, or (c) an individual can be stimulated to "interact" with other persons who are more or less far removed from him/her in space and time.

Blending the Behavioral and Interbehavioral Analysis of Interpersonal Behavior

Skinner and Kantor have much in common with respect to what is conventionally regarded in the literature as social behavior. Skinner spoke in terms of "interpersonal behavior" and Kantor in terms of "reciprogenic behavior," and both agreed that verbal behavior (Skinner) or referential linguistic behavior (Kantor) is at the center of these interactions. On the strength of these complimentary analyses, a conceptual definition of social behavior emerges which centers on the verbal-vocal and gestural behaviors of two or more people as each responds to, and is stimulated by, the other and by things and events in the environment. In elementary terms, social behavior of the sort that has captured the interest of legions of researchers over the past two decades is fundamentally a matter of someone (a child) vocally and/or gesturally referring someone else (another child) to something (a toy), somewhere (a playground) in the environment. Under the best of circumstances, we might say that the two are "having a conversation" or are "communicating with each other."

To show what concepts can be brought to bear upon an issue is an exercise whose value depends on whether the concepts have anything to do with the actual events to which they presumably relate. On the matter of defining social behavior, it is therefore important to show how Skinner's and Kantor's views are complimented by what researchers have been doing by way of "operating upon their material."

What is Taught in Children's Social Behavior Training?

Studies designed to enhance the social behavior of young children may be distinguished on the basis of their adherence to one of three conceptual approaches: Applied behavior analysis, social learning theory, and cognitive psychology. Each approach has spawned its own intervention technique, respectively, reinforcement, modeling, and coaching. Elsewhere, we have identified and discussed studies that have been represented widely in the literature as exemplary contributions to the development and refinement of the three techniques (Ghezzi, 1991). Without exception, the focus of training has been on teaching, remediating, or otherwise increasing the frequency of the same sorts of interactions that Skinner and Kantor identified as involving verbal-vocal and gestural behaviors performed by a child in relation to other people and to an assortment of things, objects, and events in the environment. In other words, what is taught in social behavior training is essentially the interactive behavior of one child appropriately referring another child or adult to some object or event in the environment.

Peer-mediation

The work on peer-mediation by Strain and his colleagues is an excellent case study of how concepts, research, and application are brought together to form a coherent approach to understanding and remediating child social behavior. To make our point, we need look no further than to one of Strain's earliest reports on peer mediation (Strain, Shores, & Timm, 1977). In that study, children with autism learned to be more socially interactive through a process that centered on teaching normally developing preschool children how to initiate and sustain appropriate play with them. Evidence for this effect derived from an observational scheme that captured all verbal-vocal and gestural behaviors that were emitted by the peer and "target" child in their dual roles as initiating or responding to an interaction (i.e., as a "speaker" or "listener," respectively). Noting that most interactions initiated by the children with autism, and responded to by the normally developing peers, were verbal-vocal, Strain et al. observed that, "Children with a limited verbal repertoire...may require specific training of appropriate verbal responses if they are to develop a complete social repertoire" (1977, p. 296).

Though not a particularly profound observation by today's standards, it nevertheless reveals not only the beginnings of an orientation to social behavior that was then, as now, on conceptually firm ground, but also an approach to intervention that takes obvious advantage of Kantor's concept of bi-stimulation. That is, given that the two sources of stimulation for a speaker initiating a referential linguistic interaction is a listener and a referent, and further, that the listener's response likewise is stimulated by the speaker and a referent, one may (a) teach the peer as a listener to sustain or reinforce the initiations of the target child as a speaker, (b) teach the peer as a speaker to evoke or set the occasion for the target child to respond as a listener to an initiation, or (c) teach the peer to assume the role as both a speaker and listener, as is typically done. When this teaching occurs in concert with child-appropriate objects and activities which supply the source of stimulation as referents, the stage is set for what has turned out to be a powerful intervention for teaching or remediating child social behavior.

It is clear, too, that the environment with and in which targets and peers interact also contains the sorts of contingencies that Skinner identified as cooperative. For instance, many of the motor activities in which peers and targets participate (e.g., sociodramatic play) appear to be reinforced on the basis of a more or less equitable and reciprocal distribution of behavior on the part of the children involved. Verbal-vocal and gestural responses may precede, accompany, or follow episodes of cooperative behavior, and may serve eliciting, discriminative, reinforcing, establishing, or even neutral functions

We mentioned earlier that one of the problems with most social skills training programs is poorly generalized and weakly maintained behavior. The peer-mediated approach of Strain and his colleagues seems to have an advantage over other approaches in that regard, and it is easy to understand why this is so. In the behavior-analytic literature on generalization, Stokes and his colleagues (Stokes & Baer, 1977; Stokes & Osnes, 1986, 1989) and others (e.g., Koegel, Koegel, & Parks, 1995) have repeatedly emphasized the necessity for "exploiting the natural environment" to achieve generalized behavior change. Recruiting and training age-peers to mediate interactions with target children under normalized social circumstances is an outstanding example of that strategy for facilitating stimulus, response, and temporal generalization. Further, there is in that same literature a consistent recommendation to "reinforce generalized responding." To the extent that instances of generalized responding occur and are reinforced under the circumstances, there seems to exist ample opportunities for a child to acquire a good deal of social behavior.

As Strain notes, the "haphazard" use of generalization strategies that accompany the peer-mediated approach are probably responsible for the generalized behavior change that he and his colleagues have found with many children. One would anticipate that future research on the approach would isolate, describe, and experimentally analyze the factors responsible for unprogrammed instances of generalized behavior change.

Future Directions

Why is so much emphasis given to teaching or remediating language in young children who show deficits or delays in it? The reasons center on the social functions that language serve, chief among them to enable a child to participate in and enjoy social interactions with other children and adults, and perhaps also, in a thoroughly unexplored realm, to interact "implicitly" with others and the "self."

Perhaps the most fundamental challenge to researchers is how to deal with certain methodological issues that arise in analyzing social behavior as here conceived. The issues reduce mainly to how to analyze the behaviors involved in speaking and listening. Steps in the right direction include (a) isolating a functionally meaningful unit of analysis, one that centers on *interaction*, and (b) developing detailed units of measurement which yield data on both the quantity and quality of social behavior.

To be sure, this will a formidable task, and one that is likely to send some researchers scurrying to the literature in psycholinguistics for solutions. That would be a mistake. Instead, we must approach matters in a way that is consistent with a natural science perspective on psychological events, taking full advantage of all the concepts, principles, and methods that have been derived from that point of view. Anything less than this will stand in the way of advancing our understanding of social behavior, and ultimately, in our ability to change behavior in personally and socially meaningful ways.

References

Baer, D. M., Wolf, M. M., & Risely, T. R. (1987). Some still-current dimensions of applied behavior analysis. *Journal of Applied Behavior Analysis, 20*, 313-327.

Chandler, L. K., Lubeck, R. C., & Fowler, S. A. (1992). Generalization and maintenance preschool children's social skills: A critical review and analysis. *Journal of Applied Behavior Analysis, 25*, 415-428.

Ghezzi, P. M. (1991, May). *Toward a definition of social skills.* Paper presented at the meeting of the Association for Behavior Analysis, Atlanta, GA.

Hake, D. F. & Olvera, D. (1978). Cooperation, competition, and related social phenomena. In A. C. Catania & T. A. Bridgeman (Eds.), *Handbook of applied behavior analysis: Social and instructional processes* (pp. 208-245). NY: Irvington.

Hake & Vukelich (1978). A classification and review of cooperation procedures. *Journal of the Experimental Analysis of Behavior, 18*, 333-343.

Kantor, J. R. (1926). *Principles of psychology.* Chicago: Principia Press.

Kantor, J. R. (1977). *Psychological linguistics.* Chicago: Principia Press.

Koegel, R. L., Koegel, L. K., & Parks, D. R. (1995). "Teach the Individual" model of generalization: Autonomy through self-management. In R. L. Koegel & L. K. Koegel (Eds.), *Teaching children with autism: Strategies for initiating positive interactions and improving learning opportunities* (pp. 67-77. Baltimore, MD: Paul H. Brookes.

Parrott, L. J. (1983). Defining social behavior: An exercise in scientific science building. *The Psychological Record, 33*, 533-550.

Skinner, B. F. (1957). *Verbal behavior.* New York: Prentice-Hall.

Skinner, B. F. (1953). *Science and human behavior.* New York: Macmillan.

Skinner, B. F. (1972). *Cumulative record* (3rd. ed.). New York: Appleton-Century-Crofts.

Stokes, T. F., & Baer, D. M. (1977). An implicit technology of generalization. *Journal of Applied Behavior Analysis, 10*, 343-367.

Stokes, T. F., & Osnes, P. G. (1986). Programming the generalization of children's social behavior. In P. S. Strain, M. J. Guralnick, & H. M. Walker (Eds.), *Children's social behavior: Development, modification, and assessment* (pp. 407-443). Orlando, FL: Academic.

Stokes, T. F., & Osnes, P. G. (1989). An operant pursuit of generalization. *Behavior Therapy, 20*, 337-355.

Strain, P. S., Shores, R. E., & Timm, M. A. (1977). Effects of peer initiations on the social behavior of withdrawn preschoolers. *Journal of Applied Behavior Analysis, 10*, 289-298.

Chapter 10

Strategies for Integration: Building Repertoires that Support Transitions to Public Schools

Patricia J. Krantz and Lynn E. McClannahan
Princeton Child Development Institute

A current theme in the education of young people with developmental disabilities is integration. Integration means that children with disabilities have the same experiences as typical youngsters. Such experiences may include enrollment in a regular preschool or school; participation in special events, such as birthday parties or trips to the shopping mall; and inviting peers to the home (Dunlap & Robbins, 1991). But for children with severe developmental disabilities, these activities may have little impact. A 1991 investigation of preschool integration (Cole, Mills, Dale, & Jenkins) found that students with more severe disabilities showed greater gains in segregated environments, and students with less severe disabilities made greater gains in integrated settings. Although imitation of typical peers is precluded in some segregated environments, there is presently little or no evidence that physical proximity of typical children and children with severe developmental disabilities results in progress for the latter.

The debate about segregated versus integrated educational settings has been clouded by the absence of sound measures of child progress. The standardized tests often used to assess the academic skills of typical children may be inappropriate for students with severe developmental disabilities (Kellegrew, 1995), and measures of progress in achieving IEP goals are frequently quite primitive. Clearly, observational measures of children's skill acquisition are immensely helpful in making future placement decisions, and we will return to this point later. But first, we will examine the characteristics of preschool children when they are first enrolled in the Princeton Child Development Institute, a specialized behavioral program for children with autism. Referred children are eligible for enrollment if they receive medical diagnoses of autism and meet the DSM-IV (APA, 1994) criteria for autism. They are not selected on the basis of IQ scores, verbal skills, or presenting repertoires.

All of the preschoolers seen during the past twenty-two years lived at home with one or both parents and, in most cases, with one or more typical siblings. They were members of families who experienced trips to parks, restaurants, and special events, as well as visits with friends, grandparents, and other relatives; thus, they were not deprived of the experiences that are important to the development of nonhandicapped children. Nevertheless, at the outset of intervention, none of them imitated others or engaged in cooperative play with siblings or peers; none appropriately interacted with parents or grandparents; none participated in family activities in the absence of stereotypic or disruptive behavior; and indeed, none displayed systematic visual attending to parents, siblings, or other persons in their environments. Before they enrolled in the Princeton Child Development Institute, some attended integrated preschools, but either they made no progress, or they were excluded because teachers were unable to manage their atypical behavior. In co-education settings, these youngsters presented extraordinary challenges. Most were not toilet trained, had little or no receptive or expressive language, and engaged in high-rate stereotypies, such as vocal noise, hand-flapping, and rocking. Some were aggressive or self-injurious. Although they were included in integrated settings, the characteristics of autism segregated them from teachers, parents, siblings, and peers (McClannahan & Krantz, 1994). Their early histories, data on their skill acquisition in a specialized intervention program, and data on their later performance in public school classrooms lend support to the importance of a continuum of educational placements for children with severe disabilities.

Programming for Integration

Given the characteristics of young children with autism who enter the Princeton Child Development Institute's specialized program, a great deal must be accomplished in order to prepare them for co-education. This endeavor requires ongoing mentoring and regular evaluation of intervention agents' skills in behavioral assessment and intervention (McClannahan & Krantz, 1994). Precise measurement of child performance permits continuing evaluation of instruction; ineffective teaching strategies are revised or deleted and replaced with more productive intervention techniques that support children's progress.

Initially, children who have little or no receptive or expressive language, and who have not learned to attend to teachers or curriculum, benefit from one-to-one, discrete-trial instruction. Such training is typically necessary in order to diminish incompatible responses, and to shape critical skills such as sitting quietly, looking at relevant materials, and pointing when requested to do so (Etzel & LeBlanc, 1979), as well as to establish vocal- and motor-imitation repertoires (Young, Krantz, McClannahan, & Poulson, 1994). But when these competencies develop, it is important to modify instruction: to intersperse discrete-trial training in a variety of other activities and settings; to introduce pre-academic and academic tasks; to provide incidental teaching (McGee, Krantz, Mason, & McClannahan, 1983; McGee, Krantz, & McClannahan, 1985, 1986); to help children learn to make choices and become more independent by teaching them to follow photographic or written activity schedules (MacDuff, Krantz, & McClannahan, 1993; Krantz, MacDuff, & McClannahan, 1993; McClannahan & Krantz, 1997) and to implement strategies to promote social interaction (Krantz & McClannahan, 1993; in press). This technology is often unavailable in regular education settings, and its absence underlines the importance of a continuum of educational placements for children with autism.

Programming Readiness for Transitions to Regular Education

When observational data document children's favorable responses to the previously described intervention procedures, it is time to assess and actively program their readiness for transition from specialized programs to co-education environments. Several objective measures of behavior, used in our setting for two decades, appear to be predictors of later success in public school classrooms.

Sustained Engagement

Ongoing attention to learning materials, teachers, and peers who are interacting with teachers is often critical to successful participation in inclusive settings. Doke and Risley (1972), Hall, Lund, and Jackson (1968), LeLauren and Risley (1972), McClannahan and Krantz (1985), and others examined the use of momentary time-sampling procedures to assess children's participation in planned activities, study behavior, engagement, or on-task behavior. Such repertoires are important because when students with autism are engaged, they are less likely to display stereotypic or disruptive behavior, and their learning opportunities are maximized. Data on the engagement of youngsters with autism, collected for more than two decades, have produced some benchmarks: when observational data show that a target child is consistently scored as engaged on 80% to 100% of time samples, he or she has met our criterion on this predictor of co-educational success.

Following Adults' Instructions

In most public school classrooms, teacher-pupil ratios do not support the presence of children who have not learned to follow directions. In fact, in regular education, individual attention is often available only because students have learned to follow individual and group directions and written instructions. Typically, teachers in regular education environments cannot provide extensive, one-to-one instruction. Therefore, measures of responses to oral and written directions, and to individual and group instructions are salient indicators of children's readiness to make the transition from specialized programs to integrated environments.

Responding to Temporally Delayed Consequences

For typical students, rewards and punishers for school performance are often very remote. For example, parents may deliver money or praise in recognition of good grades on report cards that are issued a few times per year, or may respond to poor marks on report cards by diminishing play time and increasing homework time. These temporally remote events appear to have an impact on the behavior of some nonhandicapped students, but youngsters with autism are not similarly responsive to delayed consequences without specific intervention.

In our specialized behavioral program, children initially learn to respond to the immediate delivery of tangible rewards. Next, they may earn one token and then a small number of tokens that are immediately exchanged for preferred foods or activities. Subsequently, the number of tokens needed for an exchange is gradually increased, so that access to preferred items and events is successively delayed.

When students have learned to tolerate delayed reinforcement, behavioral contracts are introduced. Teachers circle "yes" or "no" on a "school note" after each one-, three-, or five-minute interval, indicating whether the child followed instructions and completed assigned tasks, and the behavioral contract determines whether rewards are delivered or withheld. On the basis of observational data, time intervals are slowly expanded, and a youngster meets criterion when he or she performs well with reinforcement delays that encompass a significant portion of a school day. But an even better predictor of success is data that indicate that school performance is related to consequences delivered at home, by the child's parents. For example, video games or television time may be earned when a note from the teacher verifies that a youngster followed directions, completed assigned work, and did not disrupt classmates. Of course, this presumes that parents are active participants in intervention, and have learned contingently to deliver such consequences.

Exhibiting Generative Language

Typically, it takes a considerable amount of science-based intervention to help youngsters with autism acquire an initial vocabulary of tacts and mands, and to imitate others' speech. But with systematic behavioral programming, some children learn to imitate casual comments and colloquialisms, and to recombine phrases and sentences in novel ways. Our recent investigations of script-fading procedures have been particularly useful in promoting generative language (Krantz & McClannahan, 1993; in press). The presence of novel verbal responses that were never specifically trained is another indicator of readiness for a transition to regular education.

Generalization of Skills Across Settings

Often, the first step in programming for generalization of skills across settings is systematically promoting their transfer from the intervention environment to children's own homes. For example, when a preschooler with autism successfully uses the potty in the preschool, the parents visit the program and participate in the toilet routine. Next, intervention staff visit the home and assist parents with the development of a home routine; ultimately, the parents assume responsibility for maintaining the child's new repertoire, and for reporting data on successes as well as accidents. Similarly, when a child acquires a beginning expressive language repertoire, the parents first request these verbal productions in the intervention setting and later, with the support of intervention personnel, at home. The presence of parents in the specialized setting, and the presence of intervention agents in the home help to mediate generalization of new skills across settings (McClannahan, Krantz, & McGee, 1982).

Later, parents and professionals engage in collaborative efforts to program the transfer of relevant skills to community settings such as grandparents' homes, parks, barber shops, doctors' offices, and grocery stores. Generalization of functional repertoires to environments that were never the topic of training (e.g., playmate's home, clothing store, or church) is another indicator of readiness to make the transition to a public school classroom.

Low Rates of Inappropriate Behavior

Meeting criterion on the five previously described variables is sometimes, but not always associated with low levels of disruptive behavior. Although public school educators are familiar with the teasing, roughhousing, noise, and out-of-seat behavior often exhibited by typical children, a child with an earlier diagnosis of autism who displays (even infrequent) aggression, self injury, or tantrums may be reclassified or returned to the special intervention setting. Thus, a virtual absence of severe disruptive behavior is also a prerequisite for a successful transition to regular education.

On a few occasions (at parents' urging), we initiated transitions to public schools for youngsters who did not yet display the prerequisite repertoires, and these children ultimately returned to the treatment setting. During their sojourns in regular classrooms, neither their language skills nor their academic skills advanced.

Supporting Transitions to Public Schools.

In our experience, few children with autism make successful transitions from specialized programs to integrated settings in the absence of carefully planned introductions to their next environments, and continuing technological support that addresses and resolves potential problems. Such support is delivered in several ways.

Pre-transition instruction.

Teaching a child the responses that will be called for in the new integrated environment is facilitated by close, cooperative relationships between educators in both sending and receiving settings. After the next setting is identified, intervention personnel visit the target classroom to become acquainted with teachers' instructions, children's daily activities, and the materials in use, and to discuss the receiving teachers' performance expectations for the target child. Subsequently, the curriculum used in the new classroom is introduced to the child in the specialized program, so that he or she learns the academic repertoires that are expected of typical students. In addition, the youngster is taught many other specific responses: how to request use of the toilet; how to open a locker; how to articulate the new teacher's name; how to use unfamiliar physical education equipment; how to participate in new group activities; and how to put materials away (McClannahan & Krantz, 1994). This instruction not only promotes children's classroom competencies, but also facilitates peer acceptance.

Gradual transitions to public schools.

Even the most intensive intervention programs cannot instantly prepare children for all of the demands that they will encounter in regular education environments. But closely monitored, gradual transitions permit relevant instruction that contributes to later success. When a child begins a transition from our setting, he or she typically attends the new classroom for a few hours each school day, or for a few school days each week. During this time, the youngster is continuously accompanied by personnel from our intervention setting; they collect data that are later used to structure teaching activities that are provided when the child returns to our specialized program. For example, they record peers' names, and teach the child to say them. And they collect data on the engagement and social interaction of the target child and his or her classmates (see Figures 1 and 2), and use them to design additional training.

In addition, educators in the new classroom are invited to identify skill deficits and behavior problems that may interfere with the child's successful adaptation; their input is used to design special programs that support the child's expanded participation. Thus, a youngster who initially attends the new classroom for two hours per day later attends for three, and then four hours per day, and ultimately, for the entire school day.

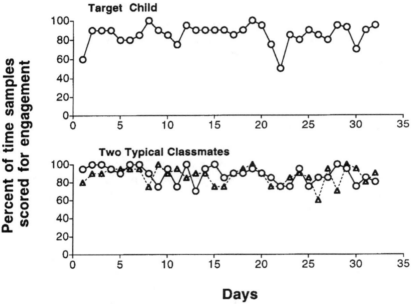

Figure 1. Percent of time samples scored for engagement in a public kindergarten classroom. Interobserver agreement on these intervention data was obtained on 10% of observations, and percentage interobserver agreement ranged from 76% to 100%.

Gradual fading of special supports.

As children's time in public school classrooms increases, the presence of special intervention personnel is gradually faded. First, an accompanying intervention agent may be stationed directly behind the child's desk; when the child is performing well, this person moves several meters away, then to the periphery of the classroom, and then to the hall. When the child's performance is stable, the representative of the specialized setting visits the integrated setting with diminishing frequency. Eventually, observations decrease to a schedule of aperiodic and unob-

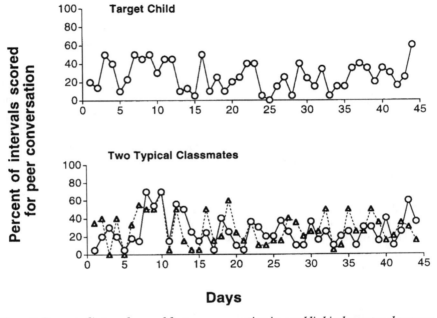

Figure 2. Percent of intervals scored for peer conversation in a public kindergarten classroom. Interobserver agreement was obtained on 11% of observations, and percentage interobserver agreement ranged from 80% to 100%.

trusive monitoring, and then to a schedule of telephone contacts with personnel in the public school. Of course, the emergence of school problems results in immediate reinstatement of classroom visits, and in some cases, regularly scheduled times for the child to return to the specialized setting for supplemental instruction. The gradual fading of special support typically extends over months.

Follow up.

Although pre-transition teaching, gradual introductions to regular education, and gradual fading of support typically achieve good results for target children, their school environments are not static. For example, when promoted to the next grade level, students encounter different classrooms, different teachers, different school routines, and perhaps even different peers. Thus, regular follow-up contacts by special-intervention personnel continue, and follow-up services remain available at the request of school personnel or parents. In some cases, no follow-up services are requested after a child achieves a successful transition; in other cases, youngsters receive follow-up services over a period of many years. Major life changes, such as the transition from elementary school to middle school, separation or divorce of parents, the death of a close relative or friend, or family relocation are sometimes associated with the appearance of school problems that can be resolved by specialized follow-up services, so that the student can continue to be successful (McClannahan & Krantz, 1994). It is a matter of concern that there are no local, state, or federal funding mechanisms to underwrite these important services.

Summary

On several continents, we have seen children with physical disabilities and children with mild to moderate retardation who appear to succeed in public schools. They participate in class activities, complete academic assignments, interact with teachers and other students, and are sometimes sought out by their typical peers. In the United States and elsewhere, we have also seen children with autism who, although they attend integrated classrooms, are entirely isolate. They attempt to engage in class activities only when prompted by teachers or aides, are unable to complete the work assigned to other students, are ignored by their typical peers, and often interrupt ongoing teaching and learning activities with noncompliance, tantrums, toilet accidents, stereotypies, aggression, and self injury.

Placing these children in integrated public school classrooms is not merely ineffective; it often produces adverse behavioral outcomes. In the typical case, staffing patterns do not permit the extensive one-to-one support that is necessary if a child tantrums for an hour or engages in ongoing stereotypies such as tapping or clapping, that intrude on the learning activities of other students. Although teachers' aides are usually assigned to such children, these persons are often poorly trained. Not infrequently, their well-meaning efforts are unsuccessful in teaching new skills, and they inadvertently accelerate inappropriate behavior by delivering noncontingent attention.

One solution to this dilemma is to radically enrich teacher-child ratios in public education, and to provide different and highly technical preparation programs for all educators, who will then be expected effectively to serve nonhandicapped children as well as children with all types of disabilities. This option requires financial resources that probably will not be allocated by government. An alternative solution is to provide an array of specialized, science-based intervention programs for children with autism that prepare them to make transitions to regular education. Measures of the effectiveness of such programs are already present (Dawson & Osterling, 1997; Fenske, Zalenski, Krantz, & McClannahan, 1985; Harris & Handleman, 1994; Lovaas, 1987).

Unlike some other agencies, our intervention program does not terminate services on the basis of age. Thus, children who meet the readiness criteria make transitions to public schools, and others may complete their schooling at the Institute and continue in the Adult Life-Skills Program, which features supported, competitive employment. Of 41 children who received services at the Princeton Child Development Institute before 60 months of age, 8 are currently enrolled in the preschool or early intervention program, 14 have made successful transitions to regular education, and 19 are enrolled in the Institute's school program. Because of the small N, the percentage of children who enter treatment before age 5 and achieve successful transitions to public school classrooms varies considerably from year to year—from 42% to 67%. These calculations do not include children who were withdrawn from the program before an outcome was achieved, nor do they include children who are presently enrolled in the preschool or early intervention programs.

Mean time in treatment for the 14 young children who successfully entered public schools is 37 months (range = 9 to 141 months). The 11 males and 1 female who are still available for follow up presently range in age from 6 to 26 years. The youngest is in kindergarten; the two oldest completed college, and are employed. Others participate in regular schools, from first grade through undergraduate school, and the majority are at their appropriate grade levels.

It is also noteworthy that, of all children served by the Princeton Child Development Institute from 1975 to the present, regardless of age at intervention, 35% to 39% have made successful transitions to public school classrooms. Although there are no comparison groups, we believe that objective measures of their readiness for transition and technical support provided during transition contributes to these outcomes.

Dependable sources of funding for these endeavors are the exception rather than the rule. Continuing research on treatment effectiveness can help to shape services, and to identify and validate relevant outcome measures. In the best case, research results will forge closer connections between program funding and children's progress.

References

American Psychiatric Association. (1994). *Diagnostic and statistical manual of mental disorders (4th ed.)*. Washington, DC: Author.

Cole, K. N., Mills, P. E., Dale, P. S., & Jenkins, J. R. (1991). Effects of preschool integration for children with disabilities. *Exceptional Children, 58*, 36-45.

Dawson, G., & Osterling, J. (1997). Early intervention in autism. In M. J. Guralnick (Ed.), *The effectiveness of early intervention* (pp. 307-326). Baltimore, MD: Paul H. Brookes.

Doke, L. A., & Risley, T. R. (1972). The organization of day-care environments: Required vs. optional activities. *Journal of Applied Behavior Analysis, 5*, 405-420.

Dunlap, G., & Robbins, F. R. (1991). *Current perspectives in service delivery for young children with autism*. Comprehensive Mental Health Care, 1, 177-194.

Etzel, B. C., & LeBlanc, J. M. (1979). The simplest treatment alternative: The law of parsimony applied to choosing appropriate instructional control and error-less-learning procedures for the difficult-to-teach child. *Journal of Autism and Developmental Disorders, 9*, 361-382.

Fenske, E. C., Zalenski, S., Krantz, P. J., & McClannahan, L. E. (1985). Age at intervention and treatment outcome for autistic children in a comprehensive intervention program. *Analysis and Intervention in Developmental Disabilities, 5*, 49-58.

Hall, R. V., Lund, D., & Jackson, D. (1968). Effects of teacher attention on study behavior. *Journal of Applied Behavior Analysis, 1,* 1-12.

Killegrew, D. H. (1995). Integrated school placements for children with disabilities (p. 139). In R. L. Koegel & L. K. Koegel (Eds.), *Teaching children with autism: Strategies for initiating positive interactions and improving learning opportunities.* Baltimore: Paul H. Brookes.

Krantz, P. J., MacDuff, M. T., & McClannahan, L. E. (1993). Programming participation in family activities for children with autism: Parents' use of photographic activity schedules. *Journal of Applied Behavior Analysis, 26,* 137-139.

Krantz, P. J., & McClannahan, L. E. (1993). Teaching children with autism to initiate to peers: Effects of a script-fading procedure. *Journal of Applied Behavior Analysis, 26,* 121-132.

Krantz, P. J., & McClannahan, L. E. (in press). Social interaction skills for children with autism: A script-fading procedure for beginning readers. *Journal of Applied Behavior Analysis.*

Krantz, P. J., Zalenski, S., Hall, L. J., Fenske, E. C., & McClannahan, L. E. (1981). Teaching complex language to autistic children. *Analysis and Intervention in Developmental Disabilities, 1,* 259-297.

LeLaurin, K., & Risley, T. R. (1972). The organization of day-care environments: "zone" versus "man-to-man" staff assignments. *Journal of Applied Behavior Analysis, 5,* 225-232.

Lovaas, O. I. (1987). Behavioral treatment and normal educational and intellectual functioning in young autistic children. *Journal of Consulting and Clinical Psychology, 55,* 3-9.

MacDuff, G. S., Krantz, P. J., & McClannahan, L. E. (1993). Teaching children with autism to use photographic activity schedules: Maintenance and generalization of complex response chains. *Journal of Applied Behavior Analysis, 26,* 89-97.

McClannahan, L. E., & Krantz, P. J. (1987). Some next steps in rights protection for the developmentally disabled. *School Psychology Review, 14,* 143-149.

McClannahan, L. E., & Krantz, P. J. (1994). The Princeton Child Development Institute. In S. L. Harris & J. S. Handleman (Eds.), *Preschool education programs for children with autism* (pp. 107-126). Austin, TX: pro-ed.

McClannahan, L. E., & Krantz, P. J. (1997). In search of solutions to prompt dependence: Teaching children with autism to use photographic activity schedules. In E. M. Pinkston and D. M. Baer (Eds.), *Environment and behavior* (pp. 271-278). Boulder, CO: Westview Press.

McClannahan, L. E., Krantz, P. J., & McGee, G. G. (1982). Parents as therapists for autistic children: A model for effective parent training. *Analysis and Intervention in Developmental Disabilities, 2,* 223-252.

McClannahan, L. E., & Krantz, P. J. (1994). On systems analysis in autism intervention programs. *Journal of Applied Behavior Analysis, 26,* 589-596.

McGee, G. G., Krantz, P. J., Mason, D., & McClannahan, L. E. (1983). A modified incidental-teaching procedure for autistic youth: Acquisition and generalization of receptive object labels. *Journal of Applied Behavior Analysis, 16,* 329-338.

McGee, G. G., Krantz, P. J., & McClannahan, L. E. (1985). The facilitative effects of incidental teaching on preposition use by autistic children. *Journal of Applied Behavior Analysis, 18*, 17-31.

McGee. G. G., Krantz, P. J., & McClannahan, L. E. (1986). An extension of incidental teaching procedures to reading instruction for autistic children. *Journal of Applied Behavior Analysis, 19*, 147-157.

Young, J. M., Krantz, P. J., McClannahan, L. E., & Poulson, C. L. (1994). Generalized imitation and response-class formation in children with autism. *Journal of Applied Behavior Analysis, 27*, 685-697.

Discussion of Krantz and McClannahan

Remarks on Krantz and McClannahan

Joseph E. Morrow
Applied Behavior Consultants

The paper by Krantz and McClannahan is in many ways a summary of their outstanding work over the past 20 years. They were among the pioneers in demonstrating, through outcomes, the effectiveness of Applied Behavior Analysis in the treatment of persons with autism.

The present paper presents some important issues. First, it raises the question of the appropriate time when autistic children should be put into the public schools. In a point that every educator and parent should attend to, Krantz and McClannahan contend that certain behavior repertoires are necessary for success. The mere proximity to the normally developing student guarantees no success and can very likely have a deleterious effect.

By delineating several behavioral criteria that appear to be predictors of a successful transition to public schools, Krantz and McClannahan have provided something quite useful for those of us who have similar programs but lack their degree of experience. One could easily rate students on the criteria they present and remediate weak areas. This could enhance our ability to successfully transition and save us ensuing problems due to overlooking some crucial set of behaviors. Essentially, the same remarks could be made about their experience based on suggestions for supporting transitions once the decision to implement them is made. Again, there are mistakes to be missed and data based steps to take to insure a successful transition.

It seems to me this paper represents the essence of an applied science. Procedures are delineated, data are gathered, sustainable conclusions are drawn and presented so that others can make appropriate use of those procedures.

Though the authors do not explicitly deal with it, the issue of the proper role of the Behavior Analyst arises from this paper. Krantz and McClannahan consider it appropriate that they try to prepare their students for integration into the public schools when such is possible. Where such integration is not likely to be successful, they try to prepare the student for "…supported competitive employment." I would argue that this is the appropriate role for the Behavior Analyst. To state it unambiguously, I believe we should use our technology to prepare our students to come under the controls that exist in the culture at large. By so doing, we separate ourselves from those helping professions that encourage dependency or do not have the technology to establish independency. Much more could be said on this subject, but it is worth noting that the Krantz and McClannahan paper is an example of this position.

Presently, the use of Applied Behavior Analysis in the treatment of autism is growing at an astounding rate. The demand appears at this moment to exceed the number of trained Behavior Analysts to do the work. With the clarity that Krantz and McClannahan offer us, this situation could possibly be remedied. Perhaps more Behavior Analysts could be induced to bring their skills to this area. Basic techniques and procedures are well spelled out thanks to such papers as the present one.